MRCP PART I REVIEW BOOK

MULTIPLE CHOICE QUESTIONS

MRCP PART I
REVIEW BOOK
MULTIPLE CHOICE QUESTIONS

Compiled and edited by
B.I. HOFFBRAND, DM FRCP
Consultant Physician and Clinical Tutor
Whittington Hospital, London.
Hon. Senior Clinical Lecturer
University College, London.

in collaboration with teaching staff from:
The Academic Centre, Whittington Hospital, London.
The Medical School, University of Newcastle-upon-Tyne.

Foreword by
J. ANDERSON, MB BS FRCP
Academic Sub-Dean and Senior Lecturer in Medicine,
The Medical School, University of Newcastle-upon-Tyne.
Honorary Consultant Physician, The Royal Victoria Infirmary,
Newcastle-upon-Tyne.

PASTEST SERVICE
Hemel Hempstead
Hertfordshire England

304 Galley Hill, Hemel Hempstead, Herts. HP1 3LE

First published 1981

Reprinted 1985

Reprinted 1987

ISBN 0 906896 03 7

British Library Cataloguing in Publication Data

Hoffbrand, B.I.
MRCP Part 1 review book. — 2nd ed.
1. Medicine — Problems, exercises, etc.
I. Title
610'.76 R834.5
ISBN 0 906896 03 7

Phototypeset by ADS, 72 Sackville Street, Manchester.
Printed by Martin's of Berwick.

CONTENTS

Brackets indicate the number of questions in each subject.

FOREWORD

Multiple Choice Questions are the most reliable, reproducible and internally consistent method we have of testing re-call of factual knowledge. Yet there is evidence that they are able to test more than simple factual re-call; reasoning ability and an understanding of basic facts, principles and concepts can also be assessed. A good MCQ paper will discriminate accurately between candidates on the basis of their knowledge of the topics being tested. It must be emphasised that the most important function of an MCQ paper of the type used in the MRCP Part I, is to rank candidates accurately and fairly according to their performance in that paper. Accurate ranking is the key phrase; this means that all MCQ examinations of this type are, in a sense, competitive.

Examination Technique.

The safest way to pass Part I MRCP is to know the answers to all of the questions, but it is equally important to be able to transfer this knowledge accurately onto the answer sheet. All too often, candidates suffer through an inability to organise their time, through failure to read the instructions carefully or through failure to read and understand the questions. First of all you must allocate your time with care. There are 60 questions to complete in 2½ hours; this means 2½ minutes per question or 10 questions in 25 minutes. Make sure that you are getting through the exam at least at this pace, or, if possible, a little quicker, thus allowing time at the end for revision and a re-think on some of the items that you have deferred.

You must read the question (both stem and items) carefully. You should be quite clear that you know what you are being asked to do. Once you know this, you should indicate your responses by marking the paper boldly, correctly and clearly. Take great care not to mark the wrong boxes and think very carefully before making a mark on the answer sheet. Regard each item as being independent of every other item — each refers to a specific quantum of knowledge. The item (or the stem and the item taken together) make up a statement. You are required to indicate whether you regard this statement as 'True' or 'False' and you are also able to indicate 'Don't know'. Look only at a single statement when answering — disregard all the other statements presented in the question. They have nothing to do with the item you are concentrating on.

Marking your answer sheets.

The answer sheet will be read by an automatic document reader, which transfers the information it reads to a computer. It must therefore be filled out in accordance with the instructions. A sample of the answer sheet, together with the instructions, is printed in the booklet of Examination

Regulations available from the Royal Colleges. Study these instructions carefully, well before the exams, the invigilators will also draw your attention to them at the time of the examination. You must first fill in your name on the answer sheet, and then fill in your examination number. It is critical that this is filled in correctly. At present, page numbers must also be filled in, but in the future, it is possible that newly designed sheets may remove the need for this step.

As you go through the questions, you can either mark your answers immediately on the answer sheet, or you can mark them in the question book first of all, transferring them to the answer sheets at the end. If you adopt the second approach, you must take great care not to run out of time, since you will not be allowed extra time to transfer marks to the answer sheet from the question book. The answer sheet must always be marked neatly and carefully according to the instructions given. Careless marking is probably one of the commonest causes of rejection of answer sheets by the document reader. For although the computer operator will do his best to interpret correctly the answer you intended, and will then correct the sheet accordingly, the procedure introduces a possible new source of error. You are, of course, at liberty to change your mind by erasing your original selection and selecting a new one. In this event, your erasure should be carefully, neatly, and completely carried out.

Try to leave time to go over your answers again before the end, in particular going back over any difficult questions that you wish to think about in more detail. At the same time, you can check that you have marked the answer sheet correctly. However, repeated review of your answers may in the end be counter-productive, since answers that you were originally confident were absolutely correct, often look rather less convincing at a second, third or fourth perusal. In this situation, first thoughts are usually best and too critical a revision might lead you into a state of confusion.

To guess or not to guess.

Do not mark at random. Candidates are frequently uncertain whether or not to guess the answer. However, a clear distinction must be made between a genuine guess (i.e. tails for True, heads for False) and a process of reasoning by which you attempt to work out an answer that is not immediately apparent by using first principles and drawing on your knowledge and experience. Genuine guesses should not be made. You might be lucky, but if you are totally ignorant of the answer, there is an equal chance that you will be wrong and thus lose marks. This is not a chance that is worth taking, and you should not hesitate to state 'Don't know' if this genuinely and honestly expresses your view.

Although you should not guess, you should not give in too easily. What you are doing is to increase as much as possible, the odds that the answer you are going to give is the correct one, even though you are not 100% certain that this is the case. Take time to think, therefore, drawing on first principles and reasoning power, and delving into your memory stores. Do not, however, spend an inordinate amount of time on a single item that is puzzling you. Leave it, and, if you have time, return to it. If you are 'fairly certain' that you know the right answer or have been able to work it out, it is reasonable to mark the answer sheet accordingly. There is a difference between being 'fairly certain' (odds better than 50 : 50 that you are right) and totally ignorant (where any response would be a guess). The phrase 'MCQ technique' is often mentioned, and is usually used to refer specifically to this question of 'guessing' and 'Don't know'. Careful thought and reasoning ability, as well as honesty, are all involved in so-called 'technique', but the best way to increase the odds that you know the right answers to the questions, is to have a sound basic knowledge of medicine and its specialties.

Trust the examiners

Do try to trust the Examiners. Accept each question at its face value, and do not look for hidden meanings, catches and ambiguities. Multiple Choice Questions are not designed to trick or confuse you, they are designed to test your knowledge of medicine. Don't look for problems that aren't there — the obvious meaning of a statement is the correct one and the one that you should read.

Candidates often try to calculate their score as they go through the paper; their theory is that if they reach a certain score they should then be safe in indicating 'Don't know' for any items that they have left blank without needing to take the trouble to think out answers. This approach is not to be recommended. No candidate can be certain what score he will need to achieve to obtain a pass in the examination, and everyone will overestimate the score he thinks he has obtained by answering questions confidently. The best approach is to answer every question honestly and to make every possible effort to work out the answers to more difficult questions, leaving the 'Don't know' option to indicate exactly what it means. In other words, your aim should always be to obtain the highest possible score on the MCQ paper.

To repeat the four most important points of technique:

(1) Read the question carefully and be sure you understand it.
(2) Mark your responses clearly, correctly and accurately.
(3) Use reasoning to work out answers, but if you do not know the answer and cannot work it out, indicate 'Don't know'.
(4) The best way to obtain a good mark is to have as wide a knowledge as possible of the topics being tested in the examination.

J.A.

PREFACE

The use of multiple choice questions is a means to a discriminating and accurate assessment of knowledge and comprehension. The Whittington Hospital and the Medical School of the University of Newcastle-upon-Tyne have, between them, extensive experience of the use of multiple choice questions in postgraduate medical education. This book provides candidates for the MRCP Part I with an opportunity to benefit from that experience.

The questions reproduce the format, and to a large extent the content of the MRCP Part I examination. However we have introduced more questions on the basic sciences in order to reflect recent changes in the exam; and the section on statistics, which many candidates find daunting, has been covered by a disproportionate number of questions.

The level of difficulty of the questions may often be somewhat greater than that of the exam itself. Please don't be afraid. Areas of knowledge that candidates find difficult have been selected deliberately. It is hoped that with adequate explanation and cross references, the questions will provide understanding and comprehension rather than be an exercise in the acquisition of factual knowledge by rote.

The questions in the practice exam, however, are aimed at the same level of difficulty as the official exam.

My thanks are due to many colleagues for their help and co-operation in the preparation of this book. However any ambiguities or errors that have crept in are entirely my own. Finally I would like to thank Mrs Shirley Low of PasTest for her patience and enthusiasm throughout this project.

BIH

INTRODUCTION

This book consists of 300 new multiple choice questions, not previously published, similar to those found in the MRCP Part I examination. Each question consists of an initial statement (or 'stem') followed by five possible completions (or 'items') identified by A B C D E. There is no restriction on the number of true or false items in a question. It is possible for all the items in a question to be true, or for all to be false.

The first 240 questions are divided into subjects and the last 60 form a complete practice exam. The subject breakdown corresponds to that of the official exam. The proportion of questions devoted to each subject also corresponds to that most likely to be found in the examination except that we have included additional questions on basic science and on statistics as explained in the preface. You should bear in mind that our subject breakdown does not mean that only questions on these subjects will be asked, or that the proportion of questions devoted to each subject will remain the same. Questions on other subjects may occur in the examination and the proportions may vary.

Answers are given to every question together with an explanation. For convenience, questions are printed on the right hand side of the page with the answers and explanations on the following page. This format is followed throughout, except for the 60 questions which form the practice exam where the answers and explanations are given at the end. The explanation for each question is necessarily brief; if you are well-informed you should find your memory adequately refreshed. If you are not, then you should seek further information from other sources. No references have been given as most students prefer to look up problem subjects in their favourite textbook.

To get the best value from this book you should arrive at an answer either 'True' or 'False' or 'Don't Know' for each item. Commit yourself before you look at the answer — this is really the best way to test your knowledge. In practice you can use the letters 'T', 'F' or 'D' to mark your answer against the question in the book. Alternatively you can prepare a grid on a separate piece of paper thus:-

	A	B	C	D	E
23					
24					

You can then mark your answers on the grid as you go along. To calculate your score give yourself (+1) for each correct item, (−1) for each incorrect item and zero for each 'Don't Know' answer.

ANATOMY

1. The foramen magnum transmits the

A basilar artery
B hypoglossal nerves
C pons
D all of the spinal accessory nerve X1
E posterior vertebral venous plexus

2. The following statements about the orbit are correct:

A the trochlear (4th cranial) nerve supplies the inferior oblique muscle
B the levator palpebrae superioris has a nerve supply from two different sources
C the superior ophthalmic vein drains into the cavernous sinus
D the ophthalmic artery is an end artery
E the inferior rectus is supplied by the oculomotor (3rd cranial) nerve

3. The thyroid gland

A is closely related to the internal carotid artery
B lies behind the parathyroid glands
C normally weighs about 30 grams
D is closely related to the recurrent laryngeal nerve on the left only
E embryological remnants may be found in the tongue at the junction of the anterior ⅔ and posterior ⅓

4. In the heart

A the pulmonary valve is normally bicuspid
B the right bundle of His divides into anterior and posterior hemibundles
C the coronary sinus opens into the right atrium
D blood leaving the coronary sinus is less de-oxygenated than the atrial blood into which it drains
E The S-A node lies in the anterior wall of the left atrium

Answers overleaf

1. D E

The two vertebral arteries pass through the foramen, only becoming the basilar artery on the pons lying superiorly. The hypoglossal nerves have their own canal (anterior condylar canal) lying just anterolaterally. The foramen magnum does, however, transmit all the cervical rootlets which ascend into the skull from upper cervical nerves, forming the spinal branch of the accessory nerve 1X. All layers of the meninges, including contents of the extradural space, pass through the foramen.

2. B C E

The abductor muscle (the lateral rectus) is supplied by the abducent (6th cranial) nerve and the superior oblique muscle is supplied by the trochlear (4th cranial) nerve. All the rest, including the levator palpebrae superioris, are supplied by the oculomotor (3rd cranial) nerve. The levator palpebrae superioris is supplied by the 3rd cranial and cervical sympathetic. Hence paralysis may be due to lesions of either. The superior ophthalmic vein is one route by which infection can reach intracranial structures. The ophthalmic artery is one of the anastomotic links between the external carotid artery (via the facial artery) and the internal carotid artery from which it arises. Its branch to the retina is an end artery. (See Q.133)

3. C E

The most important relations of the thyroid for both physicians and surgeons are both recurrent laryngeal nerves, which lie posteromedially in the groove between the trachea and oesophagus, and the parathyroid glands which usually lie in close relation to the posterior border of the gland. The left recurrent laryngeal nerve is more exposed to disease because of its long course which starts in the superior mediastinum.

4. C

The pulmonary valve is normally tricuspid like the aortic valve. It is the left bundle of His which is described as dividing into an anterior and posterior hemibundle. The heart is remarkable in that a high proportion of oxygen is extracted from the coronary blood. Hence the blood returning from the coronary sinus into the right atrium between the inferior caval opening and the right atrioventricular valve is highly de-oxygenated. The sino-atrial node lies in the wall of the right atrium.

5. Prostaglandins

A are small molecular weight polypeptides
B are chemically related to thromboxanes
C are believed to act, in part, through stimulation of cyclic AMP accumulation
D inhibit the secretion of renin
E are produced in the seminal vesicles in man

6. Plasma proteins

A migrate towards anode or cathode at different rates because of differences in electrical charges
B are mostly in the form of cations
C concentration falls early in starvation
D are involved in the transportation of thyroid, adrenocortical, and gonadal hormones
E are responsible for about 15% of the buffering capacity of the blood

7. The following have been shown to produce their effects through the mediation of cyclic AMP:

A growth hormone
B oxytocin
C oestradiol
D cortisol
E parathyroid hormone

8. Elevated serum alkaline phosphatase is a typical finding in

A vitamin D resistant (hypophosphataemic) rickets
B acute gouty arthritis
C nephrotic syndrome
D hypertrophic pulmonary osteoarthropathy
E chronic active hepatitis

Answers overleaf

5. B C E

Prostaglandins are 20 carbon unsaturated fatty acids containing a cyclopentane ring. Thromboxanes, like prostaglandins, are formed from endoperoxides. They are believed to play an important role in platelet aggregation and local vasoconstriction. The chemically closely related prostacyclin, on the other hand, is a vasodilator and inhibitor of platelet aggregation.

6. A D E

The different electrical charges of plasma proteins permit electrophoretic separation. They are mainly in the anion form contributing to the anion gap. Their weak ionization enables them to have a buffering action.

7. B E

Most protein and peptide hormones exert their effects through cyclic AMP. Exceptions to the rule appear to be growth hormone, prolactin and insulin. Thus only oxytocin and parathyroid hormone act via cyclic AMP.

8. A E

Serum alkaline phosphatase is raised in most cases of osteomalacia and rickets, but can be normal especially when the bone disease is due to renal tubular disease. In addition to bone and liver sources, elevated serum alkaline phosphatase can be of placental, intestinal or tumoral origin.

9. The following statements concerning pulmonary stenosis are correct:

A it is the commonest cardiovascular abnormality in Turner's syndrome
B the chest X-ray typically shows plethoric lung fields
C there is a recognised association with carcinoid syndrome
D an ejection click indicates that the stenosis is likely to be subvalvar
E the pulmonary component of the second sound is accentuated when the stenosis is severe

10. The following conditions are recognised as predisposing to dissecting aneurysms of the aorta:

A syphilitic aortitis
B rheumatic aortic valve disease
C Marfan's syndrome
D hypertension
E pregnancy

11. The following statements about infective endocarditis are correct:

A the most frequent symptomatic manifestation of renal involvement is a nephrotic syndrome
B the commonest organism responsible for acute endocarditis is *Streptococcus faecalis*
C petechiae are usually due to thrombocytopenia
D anti-nuclear factor is found in about 50% of cases
E the prognosis is worse when no organism can be cultured from the blood

12. In refractory heart failure

A hyponatraemia is of prognostic significance
B hydralazine acts primarily by reducing venous return
C antacids are a potential hazard
D splenomegaly is a recognised finding
E blood urea levels rise in part due to overproduction of urea

Answers overleaf

9. C

Coarctation of the aorta is the commonest cardiovascular abnormality in Turner's syndrome and pulmonary stenosis in the Noonan syndrome which has features in common with Turner's. The chest X-ray is oligaemic if the stenosis is severe, there is right ventricular failure or a right-to-left shunt. An ejection click points to valvular stenosis, as in aortic stenosis. With increasing severity, the pulmonary component of the second sound becomes more delayed and softer, and the systolic murmur extends later in systole.

10. C D E

The factors that predispose to dissection are cystic medial necrosis, which occurs in Marfan's syndrome, and increased haemodynamic stress on the aorta as in hypertension, pregnancy and coarctation of the aorta. (See Q.21 and Q.114)

11. E

The most frequently observed evidence of renal involvement is haematuria. Renal failure may develop but although proteinuria is common, a nephrotic syndrome is rare. *S. faecalis* is a common cause of subacute endocarditis, whilst *Staphylococcus aureus* and the pneumococcus are commonly responsible for the acute disease. Petechiae occur in the skin, retina and under the nails. They are probably due to immunological changes and thrombocytopenia is rare. Such changes account for low serum complement levels and positive rheumatoid factor tests but ANF is not found.

12. A C D E

Hyponatraemia is often due to diuretic therapy but occurs especially with advanced disease. Of vasodilators used in heart failure, hydralazine acts primarily on arteries, nitrates on veins and nitroprusside and prazosin on both sides of the circulation. Some antacids such as Mist. Mag. Trisil. contain substantial amounts of sodium chloride. Splenomegaly occurs with long-standing liver congestion usually with tricuspid regurgitation. Heart failure is a catabolic process with tissue breakdown contributing to uraemia and to cardiac cachexia.

13. Characteristic features of the mitral valve prolapse (floppy mitral valve) syndrome include

A early systolic murmur at apex
B midsystolic click
C a liability to infective endocarditis
D a poor prognosis
E a higher incidence in males

14. Acute pericarditis is a recognised complication of

A polyarteritis nodosa
B gonorrhoea
C thyrotoxicosis
D amoebiasis
E congestive cardiac failure

15. The following statements about atrial flutter are correct:

A the ventricular rate is characteristically about 150/minute
B an irregular pulse is a recognised finding
C DC counter shock is a treatment of choice
D quinidine alone is a recognised treatment
E carotid sinus pressure is of value in diagnosis

16. Recognised features of congestive (dilated) cardiomyopathy include

A an increased risk of systemic embolism
B pansystolic murmurs
C asymmetrical hypertrophy of the intraventricular septum
D a history of alcoholism
E a family history of sudden death

Answers overleaf

13. B C

The characteristic murmur is crescendo and late systolic. It can occur earlier in systole in some cases and is often absent. A click is a more frequent finding and is thought to represent tensing of chordae or valve leaflet. The prognosis is generally thought to be good, although severe mitral regurgitation can occur. The condition was believed to be more common in females, but the sex incidence is now thought to be probably equal.

14. A B D

Acute pericarditis is a recognised feature of all the connective tissue diseases and can complicate any septicaemia. It is a serious complication of amoebic abscesses of the left lobe of the liver. Although pericardial fluid accumulates in congestive cardiac failure, the amount is rarely significant and it is not inflammatory.

15. A B C E

The flutter-rate ranges from about 250 to 350/min and there is usually 2:1 A-V block. The block may occasionally be variable enough to give ventricular irregularity simulating atrial fibrillation. The degree of A-V block can be increased by vagal stimulation (carotid sinus pressure) slowing the ventricular rate suddenly, and making the flutter waves more obvious in the ECG. Quinidine slows the flutter-rate and increases A-V conduction. The consequence in the absence of digitalis may be a 1:1 response and a dangerously rapid ventricular rate.

16. A B D

Congestive cardiomyopathy is characterized by a dilated heart with functional mitral and tricuspid regurgitation, and congestive heart failure. Emboli are common even in the absence of arrythmias which also frequently complicate the picture. There are many causes of congestive cardiomyopathy including alcoholism, but a majority of cases in the U.K. are idiopathic, occurring in the middle-aged and elderly. (See Q.22)

Septal hypertrophy and sudden death in the family are features of hypertrophic cardiomyopathy.

17. The following statements about abdominal aortic aneurysms are correct:

A they arise typically above the renal arteries
B they are a recognised cause of ureteric obstruction
C consumption coagulopathy is a recognised complication
D the patient's prognosis is related to the size of the aneurysm
E a majority of cases present with rupture

18. The following are characteristic findings in constrictive pericarditis:

A atrial fibrillation
B normal heart size
C acute pulmonary oedema
D pulsus alternans
E third heart sound

19. The following are typical findings in acute rheumatic fever:

A apical rumbling presystolic murmur
B tender subcutaneous nodules
C cardiac conduction defects
D nail bed changes
E urticaria

20. Characteristic findings in complete atrio-ventricular (heart) block include

A variable intensity of the second heart sound
B increased ventricular rate after atropine
C collapsing brachial pulse
D regular giant 'a' waves in the jugular venous pulse
E beat to beat variation in the blood pressure

Answers overleaf

17. B C D

The majority of abdominal aortic aneurysms are atherosclerotic and arise below the renal arteries. Perhaps a majority of patients are symptomless at the time of diagnosis. Pain from the aneurysm usually means impending or actual rupture, which is more likely to occur in large aneurysms.

18. A B E

Atrial fibrillation is present in about one-third of cases. Cardiomegaly is often absent and is usually only moderate. The chest X-ray occasionally suggests considerable cardiomegaly due to gross thickening of the pericardium.
Acute pulmonary oedema and pulsus alternans would suggest myocardial disease. If, in these circumstances, there are findings to suggest constrictive pericarditis, the patient may have a restrictive cardiomyopathy.
The third heart sound of constrictive pericarditis (pericardial knock) reflects rapid but suddenly abbreviated ventricular filling.

19. C

Significant murmurs indicating carditis are those of mitral and aortic regurgitation and an apical mid-diastolic rumbling murmur (Carey Coombs) which is often associated with mitral regurgitation. Mitral and aortic stenosis only develop after months or years. Rheumatic nodules are painless. The most frequent conduction defect is seen as prolongation of the P-R interval. The classical cutaneous manifestation of rheumatic fever is erythema marginatum found mainly on the trunk and proximal parts of the limbs.

20. C E

A variable first heart sound occurs and is a sign of the asynchrony of atrial and ventricular contraction. This gives rise also to irregular giant 'a' ("cannon") waves. In acquired complete heart block, the majority of cases have a pacemaker in the Purkinje system which is not significantly responsive to exercise, vagal or sympathetic effects. In congenital heart block, the block and subsidiary pacemaker are higher and the ventricular responses more nearly normal. The arterial pulse tends to collapse as in other states with a large stroke volume. This volume and the blood pressure vary with the atrial contribution.

21. Coarctation of the thoracic aorta

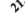

A is a predominantly female disease
B occurs characteristically proximal to the origin of the subclavian artery
C can give a continuous murmur
D is associated with bicuspid aortic valves
E has a good prognosis untreated after the age of twenty

22. In hypertrophic cardiomyopathy

A atrial fibrillation indicates a poor prognosis
B the characteristic murmur is typically loudest in the aortic area
C a diastolic murmur is present in the majority of cases
D trinitrin reduces outflow obstruction
E there are characteristic echocardiographic findings

23. The following statements about angina pectoris are correct:

A it may occur with normal coronary arteries
B it is associated with an abnormal resting ECG between attacks in about 90% of cases
C it is typically worse later in the day
D ST segment elevation on ECG is usual during an attack
E it may be aggravated by lying down

24. The following statements concerning exercise testing in heart disease are correct:

A a normal exercise test excludes significant ischaemic heart disease
B exercise testing is a useful way of assessing the severity of aortic stenosis in adults
C exercise testing may reveal significant arrhythmias
D digoxin therapy may cause difficulty in interpreting the ECG changes occurring with exercise
E a fall in the systolic blood pressure by 20 mmHg or more during exercise suggests that severe coronary artery disease may be present

Answers overleaf

C D

Coarctation occurs mainly in men. It is common in Turner's syndrome, which should be suspected in all females with a coarctation. The commonest site for a coarctation is just distal to the left subclavian artery. If the lumen is very narrow, flow through it may occur throughout the cardiac cycle. The commonest cause of a diastolic murmur is, however, aortic regurgitation due to a bicuspid valve. Left ventricular failure, cerebral haemorrhage, aortic dissection (See Q.10) and infective endocarditis are all serious hazards of untreated coarctation.

22. A E

The most characteristic abnormality in this condition is ventricular septal hypertrophy, easily seen on echocardiography. LV (and sometimes RV) outflow obstruction is variable and mitral regurgitation occurs very commonly. Atrial contraction is important for ventricular filling and gives a loud and often palpable 4th heart sound. The murmur (pan- or mid-systolic) is best heard down the left sternal edge or at the apex and is due to a variable combination of the obstruction and regurgitation. Outflow obstruction increases with trinitrin as it reduces ventricular volume and lowers arterial pressure. (See also Q.16)

23. A E

Angina with normal coronary arteries is found in cardiomyopathies, severe aortic stenosis and pulmonary hypertension, as well as in otherwise normal hearts when coronary artery spasm is often implicated.

The resting ECG is normal in 50% or more of patients between attacks. Many patients get angina on getting up in the morning and can do more without symptoms later in the day. ST segment elevation during an attack is the major feature of Prinzmetal's "variant" angina; the usual finding is ST segment depression. The mechanism of angina decubitus is unknown, but LVF and dreaming have been implicated.

24. C D E

Both false positive and negative exercise tests occur due to a variety of technical and biological reasons. Exercise testing is potentially hazardous in significant aortic valvular stenosis. This also holds for severe LV outflow tract obstruction due to hypertrophic cardiomyopathy. However, in patients without obstruction at rest, exercise may produce significant obstruction and a murmur of value in diagnosis.

25. In a patient with mitral stenosis in sinus rhythm, the following findings would indicate a severe lesion:

A long mid-diastolic murmur
B late, loud, opening snap
C soft first heart sound
D Graham-Steell murmur
E third heart sound

26. A dominant R wave in lead V1 of the ECG is a characteristic finding in

A acute pulmonary embolism
B Wolff-Parkinson-White syndrome
C left bundle branch block
D hyperkalaemia
E true posterior myocardial infarction

27. In ostium secundum atrial septal defect

A pregnancy is typically poorly tolerated
B a mid-diastolic murmur suggests a large shunt
C there is reversed splitting of the second heart sound
D atrial arrythmias are an important feature
E the electrocardiograph shows left axis deviation

28. The following statements about the arterial pulse are correct:

A pulsus paradoxus is diagnostic of cardiac tamponade
B a bisferiens pulse suggests combined aortic stenosis and regurgitation
C pulsus alternans is a sign of impaired left ventricular function
D a slow rising carotid pulse is characteristic of severe mitral stenosis
E the femoral pulses are diminished but not delayed in coarctation of the aorta

Answers overleaf

25. A D

The intensity of the first heart sound and the opening snap reflects the *mobility* of the mitral valve leaflets. In more severe mitral stenosis, the LV pressure falls below that of the LA earlier in diastole, leading to an early opening snap and long diastolic murmur. The murmur of pulmonary regurgitation occurs with severe pulmonary hypertension. A third heart sound indicates rapid filling of the left ventricle and thus excludes severe mitral stenosis (unless it is a right ventricular sound when there will be obvious signs of tricuspid regurgitation).

26. B E

Perhaps a majority of patients with acute pulmonary embolism show no ECG changes apart from sinus tachycardia and T-wave inversion over the right-sided precordial leads. S_1 Q_3 T_3 pattern, P pulmonale, right axis deviation and right bundle branch block occur, but a dominant R wave in V1 is not a feature of an acute load on the right side of the heart. It occurs, however, with right ventricular hypertrophy due to many causes as well as in WPW (type A) and true posterior myocardial infarcts. (See also Q.210)

27. B D

This is the commonest type of ASD and may well present in adult life, even in the elderly. A tricuspid mid-diastolic murmur indicates a large left-to-right shunt. It, and the classical pulmonary area systolic murmur, lessen and disappear as pulmonary hypertension develops and the shunt is reduced. Haemodynamic deterioration is often heralded by the onset of atrial fibrillation, flutter or tachycardia. Left axis deviation is the ECG hallmark of ostium primum ASD which involves the A-V valves.

28. B C

Pulsus paradoxus, a greater than the normal 10 mmHg inspiratory decrease in systolic arterial pressure, occurs in cardiac tamponade, and, less commonly, in constrictive pericarditis. It is not diagnostic of pericardial disease, but occurs in cardiomyopathies, severe asthma, superior mediastinal obstruction and shock.
A bisferiens pulse is also found in hypertrophic cardiomyopathy (see question 22), and pulsus alternans during or following paroxysmal tachycardia.

29. A 50 year old man is having treatment for pulmonary tuberculosis with rifampicin, isoniazid and ethambutol. The following statements are correct:

A the patient's eyes should be tested for evidence of retinal degeneration
B isoniazid should be stopped if serum transaminase concentrations rise
C peripheral neuropathy is prevented by nicotinic acid supplements
D treatment should be continued for at least two years
E symptoms of adrenal insufficiency may be precipitated by this treatment if there is tuberculous adrenal destruction

30. Recognised complications of vincristine therapy include the following:

A diffuse pulmonary fibrosis
B peripheral neuropathy
C inappropriate ADH secretion
D generalised pigmentation of the skin
E paralytic ileus

31. The following drugs may cause thyroid gland enlargement:

A para-amino salicylic acid (PAS)
B chlorpromazine
C lithium
D isoniazid
E phenylbutazone

32. The following drugs may raise serum thyr

A salicylates
B phenytoin
C clofibrate
D oestrogens
E androgens

29. E

Ethambutol in a dose of 15mg/kg/day as used in triple chemotherapy, gives negligible ocular toxicity, which is an optic neuropathy. Transient serum transaminase elevation is common. Isoniazid should be stopped if there is clinical evidence with biochemical corroboration of a hepatitis. Pyridoxine, with which isoniazid competes, will prevent neurotoxicity in a dose of 50mg/day. Current treatment regimes are for about nine months.

30. B C E

Vincristine can cause neuropathy, joint pain, alopecia, paralytic ileus and inappropriate ADH secretion. Pulmonary fibrosis is seen with busulphan and bleomycin and skin pigmentation also occurs with busulphan.
Vincristine (Oncovin) is part of the MOPP regime for Hodgkin's disease, and is used in acute lymphoblastic leukaemia and other lymphomas.

31. A C E

Drugs may act as goitrogens by interfering with the biosynthesis of thyroxine (T4) and triiodothyronine (T3). This, in turn, stimulates the release of thyrotrophin (TSH) by the anterior pituitary which stimulates the thyroid gland and causes it to hypertrophy. PAS and phenylbutazone have similar effects on the steps involved in the iodination and coupling of tyrosine, whereas the action of lithium is more akin to that of iodides in its effect on iodine metabolism including inhibition of release of the hormone from the gland.

32. C D

Thyroxine in the serum is nearly all bound to protein and the main action of drugs in altering the serum thyroxine is by their action on protein binding. Thus, androgens and anabolic agents lower and oestrogens raise thyroxine binding globulin (TBG).

33. The following drugs should be avoided in renal failure:

A ampicillin
B oxytetracycline
C aluminium hydroxide
D ferrous sulphate
E nitrofurantoin

34. Patients with acute intermittent porphyria should avoid

A oral contraceptives
B chlorpromazine
C sulphonamides
D aspirin
E chlorpropamide

35. Carbenoxolone

A accelerates healing of gastric ulcers in ambulatory patients
B decreases gastric acid secretion
C causes potassium retention
D may be antagonised by spironolactone
E increases gastric mucus secretion

36. Aspirin potentiates the therapeutic action of the following:

A warfarin
B probenecid
C chlorporpamide
D diazepam
E tetracyclines

Answers overleaf

33. B E

Tetracyclines, apart from doxycycline, should be avoided in renal failure as they are antianabolic, cause salt and water loss, raise the blood urea and can lead to permanent loss of nephrons. Nitrofurantoin is prone to give toxic levels and peripheral neuropathy in renal failure. It is also likely to be ineffective for urinary infections.

34. A C E

Other drugs that can precipitate attacks of acute intermittent porphyria (AIP) include barbiturates, phenytoin, griseofulvin, rifampicin and alcohol. All are metabolised by hepatic microsomes and lead to increased ALA-synthetase activity and the urinary excretion of large amounts of ALA (delta-amino laevulinic acid) and porphobilinogen in patients with AIP. (See Q.34 Page 129)

35. A D E

Carbenoxolone appears to act by increasing mucosal resistance to ulcerogenic stimuli. There is some evidence that it also speeds duodenal ulcer healing. It has an aldosterone-like action and can lead to serious salt and water retention, hypokalaemia and hypertension, especially in the elderly. Although spironolactone prevents these side-effects, it also antagonises the therapeutic actions of the drug.

36. A C

Aspirin in large doses is hypoprothrombinaemic. In smaller doses, it increases the bleeding tendency by its antiplatelet and gastric irritant effects. Also, in large doses, aspirin is uricosuric, but in therapeutic doses of 1-2g/day or less, it reduces urate excretion. Again, in large doses aspirin is hypoglycaemic, especially in children. (See Q.236)

37. Bullous eruptions are a recognised feature of

A barbiturate poisoning
B pemphigus
C prolonged chloroquine administration
D erythema multiforme
E betablocker therapy

38. Exposure to sunlight is known on occasions to aggravate

A yellow nail syndrome
B acute intermittent porphyria
C acne vulgaris
D systemic lupus erythematosus
E psoriasis

39. The following are recognised associations:

A epidermal cysts and polyps of the colon
B pseudoxanthoma elasticum and carcinoma of the oesophagus
C livedo reticularis and polyarteritis nodosa
D erythema nodosum and Behcet's disease
E skin pigmentation and the carcinoid syndrome

40. The following are recognised consequences of long-continued use of large amounts of topical corticosteroids:

A adreno-cortical supression
B skin malignancy
C a papulo-pustular facial rash
D purpura
E cutaneous striae

Answers overleaf

37. A B D

Bullae occur in about 5% of patients with barbiturate poisoning. Pemphigus is characterised by intra-epidermal bullae, and erythema multiforme by "target lesions", on which bullae often develop.
Chloroquine does not induce bullae or photosensitivity, but can give lichenoid eruptions and hyperpigmentation. The betablocker rashes are scaly and dry, not bullous.

38. D

Acute intermittent porphyria has no cutaneous manifestations. Systemic lupus erythematosus is readily aggravated by light whereas psoriasis and acne tend to be improved by exposure to UVL.

39. A C D E

In Gardner's syndrome findings may include lipomas and osteomas of the skull and jaws as well as epidermal cysts. The colonic polyps have the same malignant potential as in familial polyposis coli.
The upper gastro-intestinal bleeding that occurs in pseudoxanthoma elasticum is usually due to arterial changes.
Other associations of livedo reticularis include local heat, dependency and corticosteroids but many cases have no obvious cause.
Other skin lesions which are very common in Behcet's disease include pyoderma, papules and vesicles. A pustule on an erythematous base, occurring at the site of a needle puncture is a very characteristic finding. (see also Q.101)

40. A C D E

Corticosteroids locally give rise to skin atrophy leading to vascular dilatation, purpura and striae. The rash on the face they can produce resembles rosacea and is called perioral dermatitis. The mechanism is unclear.

41. Changes which suggest that a pigmented naevus has become malignant include

A increase in pigmentation of the lesion
B increase of hair in a hairy naevus
C ulceration of lesion
D onset of itch at site
E development of extensive vitiligo

42. The following cutaneous conditions have a recognised association with gastro-intestinal disease:

A pyoderma gangrenosum
B basal cell carcinoma
C tuberous sclerosis
D pemphigoid
E hereditary haemorrhagic telangiectasia (HHT)

43. Characteristic features of atopic eczema include

A an increased liability to develop generalised skin infection with vaccinia virus
B increased levels of circulating IgE in the blood
C an increased liability to suffer from asthma
D a positive patch test to a causative antigen
E shortness of stature in severe disease starting in childhood

44. In a patient with a rash, the finding of mucous membrane involvement would lend support to the diagnosis of

A lichen planus
B pemphigus
C chicken-pox
D erythema multiforme
E eczema

Answers overleaf

41. A C D

Other changes that suggest malignancy developing or a malignant melanoma de novo, are uniform grey or blue colour, variegate pigmentation and an irregular border or surface.

42. A E

Pyoderma gangrenosum is commonly associated with inflammatory bowel disease especially ulcerative colitis. Telangiectasia in HHT commonly affects the gastrointestinal tract and severe iron deficiency anaemia due to chronic blood loss can be a serious problem.

43. A B C

Eczema vaccinatum is an unpleasant reaction to vaccination in such patients or to accidental contact with the vaccinia virus. IgE levels are usually raised and represent reagin antibodies to many common allergens which are, however, of uncertain aetiological significance for the rash. The patients have an increased liability to suffer from asthma as have their relatives. Patch tests will not give any significant findings in uncomplicated atopic dermatitis and growth is normal unless systemic steroids have been given.

44. A B C D

Mucosal involvement is frequent in lichen planus and may be its sole manifestation: the same is true of pemphigus.
Chicken-pox often shows lesions on the palate, and less often in other areas of the mouth, the conjunctival or anal mucosa.
In its severe Stevens-Johnson form, erythema multiforme has striking mucosal involvement and cutaneous manifestations may be trivial or even absent. Eczema does not affect the mucous membranes.

45. In diabetic glomerulosclerosis

A arteriosclerosis is generally thought to play an important initiating role
B hypertension is usually the first clinical feature
C absence of diabetic retinopathy is exceptional
D nodular sclerosis (Kimmelsteil-Wilson) is the commonest histological finding
E renal amyloid may be a late complication

46. In acromegaly

A there is a recognised association with hypercalcaemia
B hypogonadism due to hyper-prolactinaemia may occur
C hypogonadism due to gonadotrophin deficiency may occur
D failure of elevated growth hormone levels to be suppressed during a glucose tolerance test is a valuable diagnostic test
E only a minority of patients have an abnormal pituitary fossa radiologically

47. In the treatment of diabetes mellitus

A maturity onset diabetes will not require insulin
B metformin is no longer used because of the risk of causing lactic acidosis
C chlorpropamide may cause facial flushing
D hyperosmolar non-ketotic coma typically requires large doses of insulin
E alkali administration is essential in keto-acidosis

48. In patients with phaeochromocytoma

A a tumour secreting adrenaline only is more likely to arise from a site other than the adrenals
B tumours in both adrenals occur in about ten per cent of cases
C preparation for surgery should generally start with a betablocker drug
D hypercalcaemia is a recognised finding
E there is an association with follicular carcinoma of the thyroid

Answers overleaf

45. C

Mild proteinuria is the first clinical feature of diabetic glomerulosclerosis and is frequently associated with retinopathy and neuropathy. Hypertension often develops later and may exacerbate the condition, but amyloid is not a complication. Nodular sclerosis, although the most specific form of diabetic nephropathy, accounts for less than 20% of renal involvement.

46. A B C D

The syndrome of multiple endocrine adenomatosis type 1 (MEA-I) involves pituitary, pancreatic islets and parathyroids and has a dominant inheritance. It would, however, be exceptional for this syndrome to present with acromegaly. Growth hormone normally should fall as plasma glucose rises, but fails to do so in acromegaly and may even rise. An enlarged pituitary fossa is described in about 90% of cases at the time of diagnosis.

47. C

Insulin may be required in a small proportion of maturity onset diabetics. Relatively small doses are usually required in hyperosmolar non-ketotic coma, some patients showing extreme sensitivity to insulin. Bicarbonate is only required in keto-acidosis if it is very severe with pH less than 7.0 and is potentially harmful because of its effect on cerebral metabolism and the haemoglobin — oxygen dissociation curve. Phenformin has been replaced by metformin because of its association with lactic acidosis. Chlorpropamide flushing, induced by alcohol, is genetically determined.

48. B D

Extra-adrenal tumours lack the methylating enzyme needed to convert noradrenaline to adrenaline and will rarely, if ever, secrete adrenaline. The basis of medical treatment is an alpha blocker such as phentolamine or phenoxybenzamine. Betablockade by itself could increase the hypertension due to unopposed alpha-activity. The tumour may occur as part of the multiple endocrine adenomata syndrome (MEA-II) in association with hyperparathyroidism and medullary carcinoma of the thyroid. (See Q.46) Hypercalcaemia is occasionally found in the absence of hyperparathyroidism or bone secondaries.

49. In patients who have been treated with pharmacological doses of glucocorticoids or ACTH

A the adrenal hyperplasia induced by ACTH therapy makes it unnecessary to give steroid cover for surgery
B endogenous cortisol production resumes when prednisone dosage is reduced to 7.5-12.5mg/day
C the potency on a weight to weight basis of hydrocortisone is 20% greater than cortisone
D steroid cover for major surgery is advisable after a year's steroid therapy however long since cessation of treatment
E rectal administration of steroids does not suppress the pituitary-adrenal axis

50. Testicular malfunction

A resulting in infertility is usually accompanied by androgen deficiency
B resulting in androgen deficiency is usually accompanied by infertility
C is the commonest cause of impotence
D in Klinefelter's syndrome will show a plasma testosterone response to human chorionic gonadotrophin
E occurs in hyperprolactinaemia

51. Prolactin

A has no established function in males
B secretion occurs in response to stress
C in excess can give amenorrhoea
D is mainly controlled by a hypothalamic releasing hormone
E secretion may be increased in primary hypothyroidism

52. The ocular manifestations of Graves' disease

A are nearly always seen when there is pretibial myxoedema
B include unilateral exophthalmos
C may occur in the absence of hyperthyroidism
D are due to LATS
E include severe pain in the eye

Answers overleaf

49. B C D

Both ACTH and corticosteroids may suppress the hypothalamic-pituitary axis. When steroid dosage approaches physiological levels, endogenous cortisol production resumes. Any patient treated with steroids for a year may have permanent impairment of his response to stress. Topical steroid administration, including rectal, may nonetheless allow enough drug to be absorbed to suppress the pituitary-adrenal axis.

50. B D E

Infertility is due to failure to the Sertoli cells to produce sperm or a "mechanical" disorder, the testosterone-producing Leydig cells often remaining intact. However, an adequate concentration of androgen is necessary for spermatogenesis. Impotence is rarely of endocrine origin or due to testicular disease. The testicular lesion in Klinefelter's syndrome is of the tubules and the interstitial (Leydig) cells may respond to gonadotrophins to produce testosterone.
(See Q.55)

51. A B C E

The release of prolactin from the anterior pituitary is largely controlled by prolactin-inhibitory factor (PIF), probably dopamine, produced in the hypothalamus. When production or release of PIF is deficient, as in hypothalamic or pituitary stalk lesions, hyperprolactinaemia occurs. Prolactin-secreting pituitary microadenomas are also a common cause. TRH (thyrotrophin-releasing hormone) releases prolactin and may play a part in the occasional hyperprolactinaemia found in primary myxoedema. The clinical features of hyperprolactinaemia in addition to amenorrhoea in women, include galactorrhoea, reduced libido and hypogonadism.

52. A B C E

Some degree of asymmetry of exophthalmos is a relatively common finding, and occasionally, it may be unilateral, especially at the outset. Loss of vision (malignant exophthalmos) may be due to increasing pressure in the eye causing optic neuritis and atrophy or corneal ulceration and severe pain may be an associated feature. Although the incidence and titres of long-acting thyroid stimulator (LATS) in Graves' disease is higher in patients with severe exophthalmos, there is no evidence that it is responsible for the eye complications.

53. The following statements regarding diabetes insipidus are correct:

A the condition is more often produced by hypothalamic than pituitary lesions
B the treatment of choice in children is chlorpropamide
C the treatment of choice in adults is DDAVP
D the absence of nocturia is strong evidence against this diagnosis
E the symptoms of nephrogenic diabetes insipidus can be improved by thiazide diuretics

54. Pseudohypoparathyroidism

A is associated with raised serum concentrations of parathyroid hormone
B is characteristically associated with an increase in urinary cyclic AMP following an injection of parathyroid hormone
C is found in the same families as patients with pseudo-pseudo-hypoparathyroidism
D is characteristically accompanied by calcification in the choroid plexus of the brain
E gives rise to tetany and convulsions

55. In Klinefelter's syndrome

A the testes may be of normal adult size
B potency is invariably reduced
C the plasma testosterone concentration may be normal
D plasma FSH is characteristically elevated
E small stature is characteristic

56. The following are recognised features of hypothyroidism:

A menorrhagia
B ascites
C cerebellar ataxia
D clubbing
E normochromic anaemia

Answers overleaf

53. A C D E

Polyuria throughout the day and night is characteristic in the untreated patient. DDAVP, a synthetic analogue of vasopressin, has an antidiuretic effect for 10 to 12 hours when administered as a nasal spray, and is the treatment of choice. Chlorpropamide potentiates ADH action on the renal tubule, but because of its primary hypoglycaemic action, is best avoided in children. The effect of thiazides is to enhance proximal tubular reabsorption as a result of causing mild salt depletion.

54. A C E

Pseudohypoparathyroidism is considered to be a failure of end organ (bone and kidney) response to endogenous parathormone, which is thus present in excess amounts. Unlike patients with true hypoparathyroidism, there is no increase in urinary cyclic AMP when parathormone is injected. Patients with pseudo-pseudo-hypoparathyroidism who, by definition, have normal serum calcium and phosphate concentrations, and patients with pseudohypoparathyroidism have in common mental deficiency, brachymetacarpal dwarfism and calcification of the basal ganglia (*not* choroid plexuses).

55. C D

Although patients with Klinefelter's syndrome have small testes due to hyalinisation of the tubules, and are infertile, some may have normal virility and potency. Serum and urinary gonadotrophins are raised. Plasma testosterone, which is produced by the adrenals as well as the testes, can be normal. (See Q.50)

56. A B C E

In addition to normochromic anaemia there is also, in myxoedema, an increased incidence of pernicious anaemia, and menorrhagia may lead to hypochromia. Fluid retention may occur, giving protein-rich pericardial, pleural and peritoneal effusions as well as dependent oedema in the absence of heart failure. An abnormality of lymphatic drainage from interstitial tissues has been implicated.

57. Iron malabsorption is a recognised feature in

A partial gastrectomy patients
B bile salt deficiency
C amoebic colitis
D terminal ileal disease
E adult coeliac disease

58. Carcinoid syndrome

A is diagnosed by detecting excess serotonin (5-hydroxytryptamine) in the urine
B may be improved by resection of secondary deposits in the liver
C flushes can be prevented by methysergide
D can lead to pulmonary valve stenosis
E can cause intractable duodenal ulceration

59. In familial polyposis coli

A inheritance is sex-linked
B the rectum is not involved
C polyps are present at birth
D there may be no symptoms until a carcinoma has developed
E about 20% of new patients have no family history

60. In the detection of serological markers of hepatitis B (HB)

A the presence of surface antigen (HB_sAg) indicates HB infection and potential infectivity to other people
B antibodies to core antigen (anti-HBc) appear before those against HB_sAg and may be the sole indication of recent HB infection
C the risk of transmission of HB from mother to child is greater in the absence of e antigen (HBe)
D surface antigen (HB_sAg) can be detected in semen
E HB_sAg positive patients with chronic active hepatitis will usually have anti-smooth muscle antibodies

Answers overleaf

57. A E

Although iron deficiency does not always follow achlorhydria, hydrochloric acid promotes the ionisation of dietary iron. Even when occult bleeding is absent, iron deficiency is not uncommon after partial gastrectomy and is also attributed to hurry and by-passing of the duodenum. When jejeunal mucosa is damaged by coeliac disease, iron absorption will be impaired, but hardly any iron absorption normally occurs in the terminal ileum or colon.

58. B D

Of the various substances produced by the liver metastases of carcinoid tumours, serotonin is the one most commonly present. However, it is rapidly metabolised to 5-hydroxyindole acetic acid (5H1AA) and it is this which is measured in the urine. Serotonin causes diarrhoea which can be blocked by its antagonist methysergide; flushing is not affected, as it is mediated by histamine, bradykinin, and unknown substances. Pulmonary valve stenosis (and tricuspid incompetence) are caused by the fibrosis induced by serotonin. (See Q.9) As the tumour is slow-growing, relief from its chemical effects by reducing tumour mass by removing secondaries from the liver, should be considered.

59. D E

Familial polyposis coli is inherited in an autosomal dominant fashion. It is not present at birth, the adenomas developing in childhood and adolescence. The whole of the large bowel is involved and carcinoma invariably develops by the age of 40 years necessitating prophylactic colectomy in early adulthood. Although 20% of patients have no family history and may, therefore, not present until carcinoma develops, the majority of patients will be detected by screening of members of affected families.

60. A B D

HB_SAg carriers are infectious, the risk of transmission from mother to child being greatly increased by the presence of e antigen. Chronic active hepatitis (CAH) may complicate between 5-10% of patients with acute hepatitis B, but is not associated with the non-organ specific antibodies occurring in other forms; again, the presence of e antigen increases the risk of CAH. HB_SAg has been identified in nearly all body fluids accounting for the different modes of transmission that are being identified. (See Q.71)

61. Hepatic granulomata

A may occur in adult pulmonary tuberculosis
B may be caused by Q fever
C when due to sarcoidosis will usually progress to cirrhosis if untreated
D when due to tuberculosis do not contain tubercle bacilli or show caseation
E usually have an appearance which is highly specific for each causative disease

62. Tests of pancreatic function show that

A secretion of bicarbonate in response to secretin is low in chronic pancreatitis
B secretion of enzymes in response to pancreozymin is low in carcinoma of the pancreas
C glucose tolerence is impaired in over a quarter of patients with carcinoma of pancreas
D faecal estimation of pancreatic enzymes is a useful screening test
E the Lundh test measures pancreatic bicarbonate produciton

63. The irritable bowel syndrome

A may follow an episode of infective diarrhoea
B does not affect the stomach
C is a diagnosis which can only be safely made following a normal barium enema
D is found to have been present in early adult life in many patients presenting with diverticular disease in middle age
E when presenting as watery diarrhoea should be treated with a low residue diet

64. The 25 gram xylose absorption test

A is usually normal in patients with pancreatic steatorrhoea
B is usually normal in patients with stagnant loop syndrome
C may give rise to diarrhoea and abdominal colic
D is unreliable in the aged
E is dependent on the surface area of the small intestine

Answers overleaf

61. A B

The cause of a hepatic granuloma cannot be determined by its appearance unless caseation or acid-fast bacilli are demonstrable, which occurs in only a few cases of TB. Q fever and sarcoidosis are amongst the many causes and the latter will only very rarely progress to cirrhosis. (See Q.107)

62. A B C

The secretin-pancreozymin test stimulates bicarbonate and enzyme secretion by the pancreas. When the Lundh test meal is administered, only enzyme output can be measured as gastric acid is not prevented from entering the duodenum. Although glucose tolerance is often impaired in pancreatic carcinoma, this is a late sign sadly reflecting the delay in diagnosis. Pancreatic enzymes are not sufficiently active in the stool to enable normal ranges to be established.

63. A

A significant minority of patients relate their symptoms, usually of painless diarrhoea, to an episode of infective diarrhoea often contracted abroad. The whole gut may be involved and gastric symptoms may coexist with colonic ones. A barium enema is not essential in all patients especially when all the typical features are present in a young person. Despite the similarities between the irritable bowel syndrome and diverticular disease, evidence is lacking that the former precedes the latter in individuals. High residue diets may be equally effective in patients with watery diarrhoea or with constipation.

64. A C D E

The absorption of xylose is dependent upon the surface area of the small intestine. Its excretion requires normal renal function and as this declines with age, the test may be unreliable in the elderly unless blood levels are also measured. When there is failure of intestinal absorption, the unabsorbed xylose may cause diarrhoea and colic. Since the intestinal mucosa is intact in pancreatic disease, xylose absorption is usually normal. The contaminating bacteria in the stagnant loop syndrome may metabolise xylose making the test unreliable in these patients.

65. In ulcerative colitis

A a complicating colon cancer is more likely to occur on the right side of the colon
B colonic cancer rarely develops in the absence of dysplastic changes in the rectal mucosa
C the main value of salazopyrine is in preventing relapses in patients who are in remission
D the rectum is not involved in a quarter of cases
E the appearance of a stricture on barium enema suggests that a carcinoma has developed

66. In Whipple's disease

A most patients are women below the age of 40 years
B fever, abdominal pain and polyarthralgia are typical features
C steatorrhoea is a characteristic finding
D the diagnosis is confirmed by jejeunal biopsy
E broad spectrum antibiotics are the treatment of choice

67. In Crohn's disease

A there is a greater risk of developing cancer when it involves the small intestine rather than the large intestine
B perianal lesions are particularly associated with ileal disease
C recurrence following surgical resection often occurs at the site of anastamosis
D about half the patients treated successfully surgically will relapse within ten years
E salazopyrine is more effective in the treatment of small bowel than large bowel disease

68. In patients with coeliac disease

A abnormal jejunal biopsy appearance may persist despite clinical and biochemical remission on a gluten free diet
B when the diagnosis has been made in infancy, a gluten free diet can usually be withdrawn at puberty
C there is a recognised association with ankylosing spondylitis
D persistent and recurrent aphthous ulcers of the mouth are a recognised complication
E the atrophic jejeunal mucosa is the result of an increased turnover of mucosal cells

Answers overleaf

65. A B C E

The risk of developing colonic cancer is greatly increased by the finding of dysplasia in biopsy of the rectal mucosa. Despite the predilection for colitis to be a left-sided disease with rectal involvement in over 90%, cancer develops more commonly on the right side. Unlike the benign strictures of Crohn's disease, the presence of a stricture in ulcerative colitis strongly suggests malignancy.

66. B C D E

This rare disease occurs in middle aged men. Arthralgia, abdominal pain, weight loss, steatorrhoea, low grade fever, lymphadenopathy and increased pigmentation of the skin are chartacteristic clinical findings. The diagnosis is confirmed by jejeunal mucosal biopsy which shows PAS positive macrophages. These are thought to contain bacilliform bodies and their disappearance after treatment with long term tetracycline correlates with clinical improvement.

67. C D

Surgery is usually reserved for cases with complications of stricture, fistula or abcess as there is a high recurrence rate within ten years. Recurrence typically occurs at the anastamosis. A complicating cancer is recognised and the risk, though less than in ulcerative colitis, is chiefly in cases with colonic involvement. Perianal disease is associated with and may precede clinical detection of colonic Crohn's disease. Salazopyrine, if of any value in treatment, is more likely to be effective in large bowel disease.

68. A D E

Coeliac disease is a life-long disorder requiring life-long gluten withdrawal. Although clinical and biochemical remission may continue after re-introduction of gluten, the mucosa will be abnormal. When first diagnosed in adulthood, gluten withdrawal may still not result in return of the mucosa to normal. Persistent aphthous ulceration may be a clue to diagnosis but there is no association with ankylosing spondylitis.

69. Carcinoma of the stomach

A is about three times more likely to occur in patients with pernicious anaemia than in the general population
B has a positive association with blood group A
C usually presents with recurrent haematemesis
D may give rise to Krukenberg tumours of the ovary
E is a late complication of partial gastrectomy for duodenal ulcer

70. Vitamin B_{12} absorption

A occurs at specific receptor sites in the jejeunum
B is accompanied by the entry of intrinsic factor into the blood stream
C when impaired in the stagnant loop syndrome can be corrected by intrinsic factor
D may be impaired in patients with significant pancreatic insufficiency
E when impaired from whatever cause will result in low serum values within a few weeks

71. Viral hepatitis

A in most cases in the UK is due to hepatitis B
B is more likely to lead to chronic active hepatitis after recovery from an acute fulminant attack than after a milder illness
C when associated with cholestasis and pruritus carries a bad prognosis
D type B surface antigen (HB_sAg) is found in about 20% of patients with polyarteritis nodosa
E may be associated with joint pains in the prodromal phase in over a quarter of patients

72. In gastric acid secretion studies in adults

A the ability to secrete acid implies the ability to secrete intrinsic factor
B the maximal secretory capacity is above the normal range in the majority of patients with gastric ulcer
C the diagnosis of a Zollinger-Ellison gastrinoma would be considered if there is more than a tenfold rise of peak over basal secretion
D the finding of achlorhydria in a patient with a gastric ulcer would suggest that it is probably malignant
E the maximal secretory capacity correlates well with the parietal cell mass

Answers overleaf

69. A B D E

Predisposing factors to stomach cancer are gastric atrophy, with its attendant hypo- or achlorhydria, pernicious anaemia, and blood group A. It may also occur in the gastric remnant after partial gastrectomy for duodenal ulcer. Occult bleeding resulting in anaemia is far commoner than frank haematemesis.

70. D

The considerable liver stores of B_{12} imply that serum levels do not fall until up to 3 years of B_{12} malabsorption have occurred. Absorption occurs at specific receptor sites in the terminal ileum where it becomes detached from intrinsic factor which is not absorbed. Malabsorption in the stagnant loop syndrome will only be corrected when bacteria have been eliminated by antibiotics. The mild B_{12} malabsorption found in pancreatic insufficiency remains ill-understood.

71. D E

Viral hepatitis in the U.K. is most commonly thought to be due to hepatitis A. Arthralgia is a common prodromal symptom disappearing, like the others, with the onset of jaundice. A cholestatic phase with pruritus does not worsen the long-term prognosis. Chronic active hepatitis is a complication of hepatitis B and can occur after a mild illness suggesting an impaired immune response of the host to the virus allowing it to persist. Other types of immune complex disease may occur in carriers of HB_sAg and the detection of the antigen in about 20% of patients with polyarteritis nodosa is of diagnostic value in this disease. (See also Q.60 and Q.215)

72. A D E

Both acid and intrinsic factor are secreted by the same parietal cells so that achlorhydria is an accompaniment of failure of intrinsic factor secretion. The range of acid secretion in benign gastric ulcer patients is the same as in normals, but achlorhydria does not occur and its presence would imply malignancy in a gastric ulcer. The stomach of a patient with a gastrinoma (ZE syndrome) is usually maximally stimulated under basal conditions and there will be little increment on stimulation by exogenous pentagastrin.

73. Prenatal diagnosis of the following inherited metabolic diseases is now possible:

A Tay-Sachs' disease
B Hurler's syndrome (Type 1 mucopolysaccharidosis)
C Lesch-Nyhan hyperuricaemia
D homozygous form of familial hypercholesterolaemia
E homocystinuria

74. The following statements concerning autosomal recessive inheritance are correct:

A if husband and wife are both carriers, 50% of the children will be carriers
B there is an equal sex incidence of the disorder
C there is an increased incidence of consanguineous mating amongst the parents of patients
D there is a tendency to "skip" a generation
E if husband and wife are both patients, 25% of the children will be carriers

75. The following conditions have an autosomal dominant inheritance:

A adult polycystic kidney disease
B Huntington's chorea
C glucose 6-phosphate dehydrogenase deficiency
D familial Mediterranean fever
E neurofibromatosis

76. There is an increased frequency of the following inherited conditions in the following ethnic groups:

A acute intermittent porphyria in white South Africans
B beta-thalassaemia in Italians
C Gaucher's disease in Ashkenazi Jews
D glucose 6-phosphate dehydrogenase deficiency in Scandinavians
E cystic fibrosis in Chinese

Answers overleaf

73. A B C E

Amniocentesis at about 16 weeks gestation is now widely used to diagnose specific biochemical malfunctions in cultures of amniotic cells, and sometimes in the amniotic fluid itself. An example of the latter is a high alpha-fetoprotein level as an indicator of a neural tube disorder. The cells can also be examined for chromosome abnormalities. (See Q.116 and Q.41 Page 146)

74. A B C

Another classical feature of autosomal recessive disorders is that only siblings are affected, the parents being clinically normal. If two patients with such a disorder produce children, they will all be affected.

75. A B E

The G6PD gene is located on the X chromosome. The majority of females are asymptomatic carriers. Familial Mediterranean fever is inherited as an autosomal recessive but there is often (perhaps 50% of cases) no family history of the disease.

76. B C

Variegate porphyria (with combined neuropsychiatric and cutaneous manifestations), is also known as South African genetic porphyria.

G6PD deficiency occurs in people of African black origin and in Mediterranean populations. The Mediterranean variety produces more severe haemolythic problems. Cystic fibrosis is especially common in northern Europeans.

77. A patient presents with urethritis and arthritis. In the differential diagnosis between gonorrhoea and Reiter's syndrome, the former is suggested by finding

A conjunctivitis
B scanty white urethral discharge
C keratoderma blenorrhagica
D pharyngitis
E necrotic pustules on the hands

78. Lymphogranuloma venereum

A is a rickettsial disease
B typically gives false positive tests for syphilis
C is a cause of penile ulceration
D may present with suppuration of the inguinal lymph glands
E may lead to rectal stricture

79. The rash of secondary syphilis is characteristically

A pruritic
B coppery red in colour
C preceded by a herald patch
D asymmetrical
E vesicular

80. False positive serological tests for syphilis persisting for 6 months are recognised to occur in

A SLE
B infectious mononucleosis
C yaws
D leprosy
E Reiter's syndrome

Answers overleaf

77. D E

Although conjunctivitis is the most frequent manifestation of gonorrhoea in infants, it is rare in adult cases. Gonococci can be isolated from throat swabs not uncommonly in gonorrhoea, with or without evidence of a pharyngitis. Reiter's syndrome is also uncommon in women and is less likely than gonorrhoea to give a tenosynovitis. (See Q. 25, Page 142 and Q.51 Page 133)

78. C D E

Lymphogranuloma venereum is caused by LGV types of *Chlamydia trachomatis*. The primary lesion is small, painless and often not noticed. Painful inguinal lymphadenopathy is the most common presentation in heterosexual men. In women and homosexual men, a proctitis is more usual. Late complications of this rare disease include strictures and fistulae.

79. B

The classical rash of secondary syphilis is widespread, symmetrical, non-pruritic, a dusky red colour and papulosquamous with a tendency to hyperpigmentation and involvement of palms and soles. Muco-cutaneous lesions are oral "mucous patches" and condylomata lata. A herald patch precedes the rash of pityriasis rosea.

80. A C D

In other spirochaetal diseases such as yaws, bejel and pinta, the serological findings are indistinguishable from those in syphilis. In many non-spirochaetal infections, non-specific (reagin) antibodies are produced, giving positive tests such as the VDRL, which may persist for years in SLE and lepromatous leprosy. Specific anti-treponemal antibody tests such as the FTA-ABS, the TPHA and TPI tests are negative in these conditions.

81. **Amongst the recognised factors impeding the rehabilitation of hemiplegic patients are**

A damage to the non-dominant parietal lobe
B mental depression
C damage to the afferent pathways
D hypertension
E dementia

82. **Incontinence of urine**

A may respond to treatment of a urinary infection
B is a feature of chronic retention of urine
C may be induced by a diuretic
D is less common in mobile patients
E is commonly due to disease of the posterior pituitary

83. **Polymyalgia rheumatica**

A is characteristically associated with shoulder girdle muscle wasting
B is characterised by a positive rheumatoid factor test
C is invariably "burnt out" after 2 years
D is significantly associated with underlying malignancy
E typically gives rise to raised blood muscle enzyme levels

84. **Hypothermia**

A is defined as a body (core) temperature of 30°C or below
B causes involuntary shivering of muscles
C may give rise to delta waves in the ECG
D is a recognised complication of alcoholism
E typically produces a systemic alkalosis

Answers overleaf

81. A B C E

Except by increasing the risks of further cerebrovascular incidents, hypertension probably has no influence on the rehabilitation of a patient with hemiplegia. The other four factors listed are all well known to impair rehabilitation. Damage to the nondominant parietal lobe may produce disturbances of the body image so that the patient is not fully aware of the orientation of the weaker side of the body or even of its existence.

82. A B C D

Inflammatory changes in the bladder mucosa due to infection, catheters, stones etc. may give urgency incontinence. In a patient whose control of micturition is tenuous, the use of diuretics will often precipitate incontinence. Any obstruction to bladder outflow such as chronic prostatic enlargement may lead to chronic retention and overflow incontinence.
Diabetes insipidus must be incredibly rare as a cause of incontinence. Far more important are the above, and gynaecological stress incontinence, with faecal impaction often playing a role.

83. None

The muscles involved are painful and stiff but not generally wasted, though wasting can occur due to disuse atrophy. It is now appreciated that the disease can remain active and need steroid therapy for many years in an appreciable percentage of cases. Muscle enzymes, as well as EMG and muscle biopsy are generally normal and unhelpful in diagnosis. The ESR is characteristically 80mm/hr or more, but by no means invariably so.

84. D

This is generally defined as a body (core) or rectal temperature of under 35°C. One of the causative mechanisms is the inability to shiver in response to the cold. The ECG changes include bradycardia and a small positive J or junctional wave immediately after the R wave. The 'delta' wave is a slurred upstroke to the R wave in the Wolff-Parkinson-White syndrome. A metabolic acidosis due in part to tissue hypoxaemia is a characteristic finding.

85. The following statements about methyl-dopa-induced haemolysis are correct:

A the direct Coomb's test is often positive in the absence of active haemolysis
B haemolysis usually does not occur until patients have been on the drug for at least three years
C Heinz bodies are a feature
D abnormal haemoglobin electrophoresis is a recognised feature
E a raised MCV is a recognised feature

86. The following produce haemolysis in patients with G6PD (glucose 6-phosphate dehydrogenase) deficiency:

A primaquine
B penicillin
C tetracycline
D glandular fever
E nitrofurantoin

87. In patients with a cold antibody haemolytic anaemia

A Raynaud's phenomenon may be a feature
B a lymphoma is a recognised association
C IgE antibody is often involved
D IgG antibodies are sometimes involved
E recent rubella infection may be relevant

88. The following are associated with microangiopathic blood changes:

A haemolytic-uraemic syndrome
B severe burns
C meningococcal septicaemia
D Down's syndrome
E typhoid fever

Answers overleaf

85. A E

A significant number of patients taking methyl-dopa develop a positive direct Coomb's test well before any active destruction of red cells take place. The haemolysis usually occurs in patients on a higher dose after 6-12 months or more of continuous therapy. There is no abnormality of the haemoglobin, either in the production of Heinz bodies or in electrophoresis. An elevated MCV is common and associated with an increased number of reticulocytes $\pm$ folate deficiency.

86. A D E

Antimalarials were the first group of drugs to be connected with the precipitation of haemolysis in G6PD deficiency. Of the antibacterial agents which can safely be given to these patients, penicillin and tetracycline are both useful whilst many sulphonamide preparations, nitrofurantoin, PAS and chloramphenicol precipitate haemolysis. Many viral infections precipitate haemolysis in G6PD deficiency and glandular fever is a good example of this. (See also Q.75 and Q.76)

87. A B D E

Raynaud's phenomenon occurs when cold antibodies cause in vivo agglutination at the cold peripheries. These antibodies are usually IgM or IgG in class and the IgM are often associated with lymphoma. The Donath-Landsteiner IgG cold antibody was, in the past, commonly seen with syphilis, but now viral infections such as rubella are the most frequent cause.

88. A B C

Fragmented red cells are seen in the haemolytic-uraemic syndrome and the closely related thrombotic thrombocytopenic purpura. The destruction of small superficial vessels by burns causes breaking up of the red cells as they pass through. In meningococcal sepsis the microangiopathy can be associated with DIC. Microangiopathic anaemia occurs in other conditions with DIC such as septic shock and in malignant hypertension and polyarteritis nodosa.

89. Idiopathic thrombocytopenic purpura (ITP)

A in adults frequently follows a viral infection
B in childhood is characteristically complicated by extensive haemorrhages and a fulminant course
C is characteristically associated with moderate splenomegaly
D is known to occur in children born to a mother previously cured of ITP by splenectomy
E is associated with a reduction of megakaryocytes on bone marrow examination

90. In the investigation of a patient with a bleeding tendency

A a prolonged partial thromboplastin time could indicate haemophilia
B a normal prothrombin time excludes thrombocytopenia
C haemophilia and Xmas disease can be distinguished by a thromboplastin generation test
D Hess' test is negative with a coagulation factor deficiency
E a prolonged prothrombin time is a characteristic finding in hereditary haemorrhagic telangiectasia (HHT)

91. In beta-thalassaemia major

A symptoms and signs typically develop at about five years of age
B in children, there is seldom marked enlargement of the spleen
C the mongoloid facies is due to expansion of the facial bones due to marrow hyperplasia
D the serum iron is often raised although the MCH is reduced
E the anaemia is entirely due to decreased haemoglobin synthesis

92. Macrocytosis of red cells is a recognised finding in

A coeliac disease
B ulcerative colitis
C alcoholism
D aplastic anaemia
E patients treated with methotrexate

Answers overleaf

89. D

ITP in childhood often follows viral infection, but in adults, the onset is usually more insidious. Most cases resolve spontaneously in childhood, and the patients do not have splenomegaly. Even though the mother may be clinically "cured" by splenectomy, circulating antibodies may still be present and can affect the baby at the time of delivery. In ITP, megakaryocytes are normal or increased in the marrow. (See Q.98)

90. A C D

The partial thromboplastin time is prolonged with deficiencies of the intrinsic system factors V111 and 1X which do not affect the prothrombin time. The prothrombin time is prolonged with deficiency of the extrinsic system factor V11 as well as the common pathway factors X, V and II. Hess' test is abnormal with small vessel abnormality, thrombocytopenia and impaired platelet function. The bleeding disorder in HHT is due to the abnormal mucosal blood vessels. (See Q.100 and Q.27 Page 142)

91. C D

In severe thalassaemia major, symptoms and signs develop in the first two years of life and marked enlargement of the spleen is very common. Mongoloid facies are typical of all the congenital haemolytic anaemias in which there is marked marrow hyperplasia. Raised serum iron occurs with iron therapy, haemochromatosis, sideroblastic anaemia and the thalassaemias. In beta-thalassaemia major, there is significant under-haemoglobinisation of red cells associated with a very low MCH. The anaemia is due to a combination of ineffective erythropoiesis and haemolysis.

92. A C D E

The macrocytosis of coeliac disease is usually due to folate deficiency. Alcohol makes the red cells large directly, through secondary folate deficiency and with liver disease. In aplasia, younger large red cells are thrown out from the marrow. Methotrexate causes megaloblastic change due to folate antagonism. A reticulocytosis is also a cause of macrocytosis.

93. Pancytopenia may be caused by

A folic acid deficiency
B paroxysmal nocturnal haemoglobinuria (PNH)
C miliary tuberculosis
D acute myeloblastic leukaemia
E haemosiderosis

94. Blood eosinophilia is a recognised feature of

A Hodgkin's disease
B malaria
C polyarteritis nodosa
D systemic lupus erythematosus
E farmer's lung

95. The following are recognised complications of Hodgkin's disease:

A amyloidosis
B dermatomyositis
C cryptococcus infection
D haemolytic anaemia
E asthma

96. As compared with chronic myelocytic leukaemia, chronic lymphocytic leukaemia has

A more marked lymphadenopathy
B more frequent hypogammaglobulinaemia
C a more frequent occurrence of a positive Coomb's test
D more frequent development of a blast crisis
E a worse prognosis

Answers overleaf

93. A B C D

Important causes of pancytopenia which are potentially reversible also include vitamin B_{12} deficiency, SLE, hypersplenism, and drug-induced marrow aplasia.

94. A B C

Protozoal infections such as malaria tend not to give eosinophilia as frequently as many parasitic infestations. Eosinophilia commonly occurs with a variety of allergic disorders such as asthma, eczemas and drug reactions. It is also a feature of a number of rare conditions with extensive tissue infiltration presenting with cardiomyopathy, a scleroderma-like syndrome (eosinophilic fasciitis), gastrointestinal disease or pulmonary disease.

95. A C D

There is a T-cell defect in Hodgkin's disease which reflects the long-standing observation of cutaneous anergy in this condition. This probably explains the predisposition to certain infections such as TB, cryptococcosis, toxoplasmosis, pneumocystis, aspergillosis, herpes zoster and disseminated varicella. Treatment undoubtedly aggravates the predisposition.
Haemolytic anaemia is much rarer in Hodgkin's disease than with lymphocytic neoplasia.

96. A B C

Patients with chronic lymphocytic leukaemia also tend to be older, the splenomegaly is not as marked, and is painful much less often. Auto-immune thrombocytopenia also can complicate CLL, though less frequently than an auto-immune haemolytic anaemia

97. Features of sickle cell anaemia in adults include

A leg ulcers
B aseptic bone necrosis
C dysphagia
D priapism
E nocturia

98. Immune mechanisms are believed to be responsible for thrombocytopenia due to

A pernicious anaemia
B alcohol
C idiopathic thrombocytopenic purpura
D systemic lupus erythematosus
E disseminated intravascular coagulation

99. In the differential diagnosis of a raised haematocrit, the following suggest polycythaemia rubra vera:

A low serum B_{12}
B high serum iron
C normal white cell count
D splenomegaly
E reduced number of bone marrow megakaryocytes

100. The bleeding disorder in the following conditions is due primarily to thrombocytopenia:

A von Willebrand's disease
B quinidine sensitivity
C Goodpasture's syndrome
D oxyphenbutazone therapy
E scurvy

Answers overleaf

97. A B D E

Infection of bone infarcts occurs and tends to be with salmonella. Other problems of the adult sickler include severe anaemia, crises, pulmonary infarcts, gallstones, cerebrovascular complications and recurrent haematuria.

98. C D

Vitamin B_{12} (and folate) deficiency causes thrombocytopenia by interfering with megakaryocyte maturation, alcohol by marrow suppression and DIC by increased consumption. (See Q.89)

99. D

In the classical case, evidence of increased production of all the marrow elements and splenomegaly distinguishes polycythaemia rubra vera from secondary and relative ("stress") polycythaemia. The serum iron tends to be low and the serum B_{12} high due to an increase in the vitamin B_{12} binding proteins.

100. B D

In von Willebrand's disease, the bleeding disorder is due to a deficiency of von Willebrand's factor, a part of factor VIII which is needed for platelet adhesion to endothelium. (See Q.90 and Q.27 Page 142) In Goodpasture's syndrome and scurvy, the abnormal bleeding is due to loss of capillary integrity. Quinidine produces thrombocytopenia by an immunological mechanism, and oxyphenbutazone by megakaryocyte or pan-marrow suppression.

101. Characteristic features of Behçet's disease include

A thrombophlebitis
B glomerulonephritis
C scrotal ulceration
D pyoderma gangrenosum
E myocarditis

102. The following have a recognised association with IgM paraprotein:

A kala-azar
B cold haemagglutinin disease
C chronic lymphatic leukaemia (CLL)
D Waldenstrom's disease
E chronic myeloid leukaemia

103. The serum sickness reaction in clinical practice

A is believed to involve complement activation
B causes a progressive glomerulonephritis
C usually responds to the administration of systemic steroids
D leads to inflammation of small blood vessels
E typically appears about 48 hours after the administration of serum

104. Characteristic features of common variable immunodeficiency (idiopathic hypogammaglobulinaemia) include

A splenomegaly
B bronchiectasis
C pernicious anaemia
D *Giardia lamblia* infestation
E recurrent viral hepatitis

Answers overleaf

101. A C

Arthritis, anterior uveitis and CNS involvement are other characteristic features. Skin lesions, pustules, papules and erythema nodosum, are common. (See Q.39 and Q.138)

102. B C D

No paraproteins are seen in kala-azar, but often there is a massive polyclonal rise in IgM. Cold agglutinin disease, CLL, Waldenstrom's disease, are all B-cell lymphoproliferative disorders sometimes associated with an IgM paraprotein, whilst this is not seen in any of the myeloproliferative disorders.

103. A C D

Serum sickness is due to immune complex deposition with complement activation. Vasculitis is prominent and accounts for the major features of fever, rashes, oedema, arthralgia and a mild non-progressive glomerulonephritis. Symptoms occur at the time of the antibody response about one week or more after antigen exposure.

104. A B C D

Lymphoid tissue hyperplasia is a typical finding amongst this group of patients who have the most frequent form of primary immunodeficiency. Recurrent pneumonia (leading to bronchiectasis), sinusitis, otitis media, and gastrointestinal infections are the most frequent infections. There is no marked predisposition to recurrent viral infections. There is, however, a high incidence, remarkably, of autoimmune disorders.

105. Glandular fever-like syndromes may result from infection with

A *Toxoplasma gondii*
B herpes simplex type 2
C cytomegalovirus
D Epstein-Barr virus
E echovirus 19

106. Chlamydia trachomatis

A is characteristically associated with HLA-B27 positive patients
B is a cause of non-specific urethritis
C gives neonatal eye infections which are clinically indistinguishable from gonococcal eye infections
D causes lymphogranuloma venereum
E gives eye infections which are treated with chloramphenicol by preference

107. Q Fever

A is caused by *Coxiella burnetii*
B is an occupational disease
C is diagnosed by blood culture
D commonly gives pneumonitis
E responds well to penicillin therapy

108. Characteristic findings in acquired toxoplasmosis include

A cervical lymphadenopathy
B polymorph leucocytosis
C exudative pharyngitis
D autoimmune haemolytic anaemia
E anterior uveitis

Answers overleaf

105. A C D

Glandular fever-like syndromes can be caused by toxoplasmosis, (See Q.108), cytomegalovirus, and the Epstein-Barr virus (EBV). Infectious mononucleosis (glandular fever) is caused specifically by the Epstein-Barr virus: the Paul-Bunnell test measures heterophil antibody and may be negative in the presence of EBV antibody.

106. B C D

Chlamydia trachomatis is associated with sero-negative arthritis but not especially with HLA-B27 positive patients. Chlamydia is one of the causes of "non-specific urethritis", but technically it is now a specific cause of urethritis. The treatment of choice is topical tetracycline and systemic erythromycin.

107. A B D

This rickettsial disease occurs in animal and animal-product handlers. Pneumonitis and a granulomatous hepatitis are common manifestations. Endocarditis is a rare one. The diagnosis is serological and treatment is with tetracycline antibiotics. (See Q.61)

108. A

The most frequent manifestation of acquired toxoplasmosis is lymphadenopathy, especially cervical. With malaise and atypical lymphocytes, the picture often resembles glandular fever. (See Q.105) Isolated anterior uveitis does not occur in the acquired disease. Choroidoretinitis, a characteristic feature of congenital toxoplasmosis, does, however, occasionally develop.

109. Characteristic features of brucellosis include

A leucocytosis
B spondylitis
C marked sweating
D pruritus
E mental depression

110. Rigors are a typical feature of

A brucellosis
B acute pyelonephritis
C typhoid
D acute cholangitis
E pulmonary tuberculosis

111. Characteristic features of the first week of typhoid fever include

A delirium
B intestinal haemorrhage
C headache
D leucocytosis
E positive blood cultures

112. In diphtheria

A the membrane is confined to the tonsils
B cervical adenopathy is a characteristic finding
C fever over 40°C is usually present
D a bloody nasal discharge is a recognised finding
E myocarditis typically has a good prognosis

Answers overleaf

109. B C E

A majority of the symptoms of brucellosis are non-specific and associated with fever, but septicaemic complications such as osteomyelitis of the spine, arthritis and endocarditis can occasionally occur. A white cell count over $10{,}000/mm^3$ would make the diagnosis suspect.

110. A B D

A true rigor, which is bed-shaking, is characteristic of pyogenic infections with bacteraemia, and other infections such as malaria. True rigor can also occur with viraemia. Perhaps the majority of cases of brucellosis have a more gradual onset. (See Q.109)

111. C E

Prominent symptoms in the early phase of typhoid fever are headache, malaise, anorexia, constipation and a dry cough. A leucopenia is a characteristic finding in typhoid fever. A leucocytosis would suggest some complication such as intestinal perforation.

112. B D

A membrane is not invariable, but can be situated in the pharynx or nasal passages and can extend to occlude the larynx. High fever would suggest a superadded infection with a group A *Streptococcus pyogenes*. (See Q.43 Page 146)

113. Hypophosphataemic rickets ("vitamin D resistant") is characterised by

A an autosomal recessive inheritance
B excessive renal tubular loss of phosphate
C short stature
D calcification of inter-spinous ligaments
E complete resistance to treatment by vitamin D

114. The following features of Marfan's disease distinguish it from homocystinuria:

A autosomal dominant inheritance
B lens dislocation
C joint laxity
D rupture of aortic aneurysm
E arachnodactyly

115. The following are recognised findings in osteogenesis imperfecta:

A blue sclerae
B otosclerosis
C pathological fracture
D low alkaline phosphatase
E partial remission in the female reproductive years

116. Hyperuricaemia is a recognised consequence of

A hypercalcaemia
B cyanotic heart disease
C Hypoxanthine-guanine-phosphoribosyl transferase (HGPRT) deficiency
D inhibition of xanthine oxidase
E glucose-6-phosphatase deficiency (Type I glycogen storage disease)

Answers overleaf

113. B C D

Hypophosphataemic rickets is characterised by an X-linked dominant inheritance and affects both males and females. Whereas an excessive tubular loss of phosphate is considered to be the fundamental cause of the condition, it is possible that there is an increased gastro-intestinal loss. Treatment is based on giving large doses of vitamin D together with phosphate supplements, but even with treatment from an early age, it is not thought that normal stature will be obtained. Some cases present in adult life. Calcification of interspinous ligaments occurs, sometimes confused with ankylosing spondylitis or hyperostosis.

114. A C D

Homocystinuria is often wrongly diagnosed as Marfan's syndrome on account of some clinical similarities, but can readily be distinguished by a positive cyanide-nitroprusside test on urine for homocystine and more specifically by finding an excess of homocystine and methionine on blood and urine chromatography. Homocystinuria has an autosomal recessive inheritance and no evidence of joint laxity. Whereas Marfan's patients may suffer aortic dilatation and rupture, (See Q.10) and mitral regurgitation, homocystinurics have no specific cardiac defects but do have a general thrombotic tendency which may cause myocardial, pulmonary or cerebral infarction.

115. A B C E

Osteogenesis imperfecta, in which there appears to be a generalised defect in the maturation of collagen, manifests in the eye (blue sclerae), ear (otosclerosis), skeleton (multiple fractures), loose jointedness and in skin. The alkaline phosphatase is normal or perhaps raised following a fracture. There is said to be a partial remission from pathological fractures during the reproductive years in women presumably owing to the effects of oestrogen. A low alkaline phosphatase is characteristic of hypophosphatasia, a rare inherited syndrome of short stature, which usually presents as rickets.

116. A C E

Hypercalcaemia giving renal failure or due to hyperparathyroidism is associated with hyperuricaemia. Polycythaemia and other myelo- and lymphoproliferative diseases give overproduction of uric acid. Deficiency of HGPRT is the cause of the Lesch-Nyhan syndrome (See Q.73) in which gross over-production of uric acid is associated with choreoathetosis, spasticity, variable mental deficiency and self-mutilation. Children with type I glycogen storage disease develop gout as a consequence of impaired uric acid excretion secondary to lactic acidosis and ketonaemia, and increased de novo purine synthesis. Xanthine oxidase inhibitors such as allopurinol lower blood urate levels.

117. Staphylococci

A are gram-positive spherical motile organisms
B are arranged in chains
C are facultative anaerobes
D do not produce an exotoxin
E produce coagulase

118. The following statements about *Escherichia coli* are correct:

A many of the strains are not pathogenic
B it is a non-lactose fermenter
C it characteristically gives rise to foul smelling infections
D it has a recognisable appearance on gram stain
E it grows anaerobically

119. *Mycobacterium tuberculosis*

A does not grow well anaerobically
B produces pigmented colonies on exposure to light
C resists decoloration with acid-alcohol after staining with carbolfuchsin
D is non-motile
E is distinguished from *M. leprae* in culture media by the relative rates of colony growth

120. *Clostridium tetani*

A is pathogenic by virtue of an endotoxin
B is gram-negative
C bears spores
D is sensitive to tetracycline
E is highly resistant to antiseptics

Answers overleaf

117. C E

Staphylococci are not motile, grow in clusters, are coagulase-positive, and although aerobic, tolerate an anaerobic atmosphere quite well. Some strains produce an exotoxin called enterotoxin responsible for one form of food poisoning. An exotoxin is also produced by some strains which produces shock. It has been implicated in human disease, most recently in cases of the tampon-associated toxic shock syndrome.

118. E

E. coli belong to the Enterobacteriaceae which include *Salmonella, Shigella* and *Proteus* (non lactose-fermenters) and *Klebsiella, Enterobacter* and others (lactose-fermenters). All the strains are potential pathogens; foul-smelling pus indicates anaerobes such as *Bacteroides* with which *E. coli* may well be associated. The microscopic appearances are not characteristic and biochemical and serological tests are needed for differentiation from other enterobacteria.

119. A C D

M. tuberculosis is a strict aerobe growing especially well in enviroments with a high pO_2 such as lung, kidney and skin. The "acid-fastness" is related to the integrity of the waxy cell-wall. The colonies of one group of "atypical" mycobacteria, but not tubercle bacilli, go yellow after brief exposure to light. At the time of going to press *M. leprae* had not been cultured in artificial media!

120. C D

C. tetani gives clinical effects by means of an exotoxin, tetanospasmin (tetanus toxin). The bacilli are gram-positive and are spore-bearing; the spores give the bacillus a "drum-stick" or "dumb-bell" appearance. The spores are resistant to antiseptics, drying and to a degree, to heat but the bacilli themselves are not. Although they are sensitive to tetracycline, penicillin is probably the antibiotic of choice.

121. A lesion which involves the right half of the eighth cervical segment of the spinal cord may

A impair position sense in the right leg
B abolish the right biceps reflex
C abolish the right abdominal reflexes
D impair pain and temperature sensibility below the level of the lesion on the right side
E cause clonus at the right ankle

122. Characteristic features of occlusion of the left middle cerebral artery include

A a hemiplegia that affects the leg more than the arm
B paralysis of conjugate gaze towards the left
C deep xanthochromia of the cerebrospinal fluid
D diplopia
E dementia

123. Chorea is a recognised complication of

A oral contraceptive agents
B chlorpromazine
C L-dopa
D benserazide hydrochloride
E cholestyramine

124. The anterior horn cells show pathological changes in

A botulism
B tetanus
C the progressive muscular atrophy type of motor neurone disease
D Refsum's disease
E anterior spinal artery thrombosis

Answers overleaf

121. A C E

Position sense is mediated by the posterior columns which do not cross in the cord. The pyramidal lesion will similarly affect the right side.

122. None

The motor and sensory abnormalities vary depending on the exact site of occlusion, but occur mainly in the face and upper extremities. Other findings in this case might be dysphasia and right homonymous hemianopia.

123. A C

The mechanism whereby chorea is caused by oral contraceptive agents has not been clarified. It is commoner in patients who have had Sydenham's chorea and may be due to altered sensitivity of the dopaminergic receptors.

Excessive dopaminergic activity by L-dopa induces chorea, and aggravates the abnormal movements of Huntington's chorea.

124. C E

The predominant lesion in the progressive muscular atrophy type of motor neurone disease is degeneration of the anterior horn cells. The anterior spinal artery sends off circumflex branches around the outside of the spinal cord. These in turn give rise to perforating branches which directly supply the anterior horns, so this area may be infarcted.

125. Complications of phenytoin therapy include

A bulbar palsy
B megaloblastic anaemia
C hirsutism
D menstrual irregularity
E urinary retention

126. The following are recognised presentations of a pituitary chromophobe adenoma:

A CSF rhinorrhoea
B binasal visual field defect
C anorexia nervosa
D petit mal epilepsy
E sudden monocular blindness

127. Pseudo-bulbar palsy

A may be caused by multiple sclerosis
B is associated with a grasp reflex
C is associated with emotional incontinence
D is typically associated with impairment of intellectual function
E responds to tetrabenazine

128. Diabetic amyotrophy

A affects predominantly the distal muscles of the lower limbs
B is associated with elevated CSF protein levels
C usually responds to improved control of blood sugar levels
D causes impotence
E causes urinary retention

Answers overleaf

125. B C D

Hirsutism and coarsening of facial features make phenytoin a drug to be avoided if possible in young people. The megaloblastic anaemia is folate-responsive. Other side-effects of chronic usage include a cerebellar syndrome, gum hypertrophy, rashes, liver disease and peripheral neuropathy.

126. A B C E

A pituitary tumour may erode the dura and bone of the sella turcica into the sphenoidal air sinus and cause CSF rhinorrhoea and recurrent meningitis. Any visual field defect may occur from chiasmal compression and distortion. Although temporal defects are commonest, nasal loss is more likely when the chiasm is prefixed and distorted so that maximum damage is done anteriorly. Psychological disturbances occur from hypothalamic involvement and monocular blindness from pressure on the blood supply to the optic nerve.

127. A C

Pseudo-bulbar palsy is caused by bilateral lesions of the upper motor neurone tracts in the brain stem. Multiple sclerosis is a common cause in young adults.
The association of emotional incontinence with pseudo-bulbar palsy is related to the rostral extension of the pathological process to involve connections with the frontal lobes.

128. B C

Diabetic amyotrophy causes demyelination in the lumbar and cervical roots resulting in pain, weakness and wasting in proximal limb muscles.
Improved control of blood sugar levels usually results in recovery, which is not the case with other forms of diabetic peripheral neuropathy.

129. Absent ankle jerks are associated with extensor plantar responses in

A tabes dorsalis
B vitamin B_{12} deficiency
C amyotrophic lateral sclerosis
D lesions of the conus medullaris
E dorsal disc protrusion

130. There is a known association between chronic alcoholism and

A proximal myopathy
B auditory hallucinosis
C Purkinje cell atrophy in the cerebellum
D pendular nystagmus
E hypoglycaemia

131. Acoustic neuroma

A causes facial palsy in about 60% of cases
B may present with trigeminal neuralgia
C has an association with phaeochromocytoma
D has an association with occipital muscle spasm
E causes bulbar palsy

132. Polymyositis

A is associated with thymoma
B may result in pseudo-hypertrophy of muscle
C may result in subcutaneous calcification in children
D may result in myoglobulinuria
E has a good prognosis in children

Answers overleaf

129. B D

Deficiency of vitamin B_{12} causes degeneration of the posterior columns of the spinal cord and a peripheral neuropathy. This interferes with the afferent part of the reflex arc. The degeneration of the lateral columns results in extensor plantar responses.
In the conus medullaris, the sacral root entry zones and anterior horn cells are crowded together and in close proximity to the pyramidal tracts. A relatively small lesion in this area may thus cause upper and lower motor neurone signs in the lower limbs. Taboparesis and Friedreich's ataxia may also produce these signs.

130. A B C E

Painful, acute, and chronic proximal myopathy occurs in alcoholics. Auditory hallucinosis is one of the specific withdrawal syndromes.
Cerebellar Purkinje cell atrophy may occur as part of multiple CNS damage or as an entity. Pendular nystagmus occurs with visual defects. Hypoglycaemia is believed to result from the blockage of gluconeogenesis when there are depleted liver glycogen stores. Children are especially prone to alcohol-induced hypoglycaemia. (See also Q.172)

131. B C D E

About 15% of acoustic neuroma are associated with facial palsy. During the irritative phase, trigeminal neuralgia may occur, but this gives way to loss of trigeminal sensory function. Phaeochromocytoma is associated with neurofibromatosis in which bilateral acoustic neuromas occur. Irritation of the surrounding dura may cause occipital muscle spasm (Cairn's sign). As the tumour grows, the fifth, seventh, ninth, tenth, eleventh and twelfth cranial nerves become involved; with pressure on the brain stem, the contralateral nerves become distorted.

132. A B C D E

Polymyositis in adults is associated in 10% or more cases with many types of malignancy. The chronic form of the disease may result in pseudo-hypertrophy of skeletal muscle as fibrous tissue is laid down. The mechanism of calcification in the dermis in children is not known. The acute and sometimes massive destruction of muscle leads to leakage of myoglobin and may result in renal failure. Polymyositis in children is usually acute and responds well to steroids.

133. Unilateral ptosis is a recognised finding in

A syringobulbia
B cluster headaches
C Bell's palsy
D cavernous sinus syndrome
E tabes dorsalis

134. In subarachnoid haemorrhage from a ruptured aneurysm

A the risk of further haemorrhage is greatest after four weeks
B the control of hypertension may influence the prognosis
C fever is common
D internal hydrocephalus may be a late complication
E Korsakoff's psychosis may be a late complication

135. Parkinsonism is a recognised complication of treatment with

A reserpine
B magnesium salts
C perphenazine
D haloperidol
E dexamethasone

136. Neuropathic joints are a recognised complication of

A Huntington's chorea
B syringomyelia
C amyotrophic lateral sclerosis
D diabetes mellitus
E leprosy

Answers overleaf

133. A B D E

Syringobulbia damages the sympathetic pathways of the medulla. Cluster headaches result from acute dilatation of arterioles in the distribution of the external carotid artery with oedema and ischaemia of the accompanying sympathetic nerves. This is particularly severe in the periorbital vasculature. Pathology in the cavernous sinus interferes with nerve function and the levator palpebrae muscle may be partially denervated. (See Q.2)

Tabes dorsalis causes fibrosis from endarteritis in the sympathetic chains.

134. B C D E

The risk of further haemorrhage rises to a peak at 10 days. It has been shown that control of the diastolic blood pressure to about 100 mmHg improves the prognosis, whether the hypertension is long-standing or the result of the intracranial event.

Any foreign material in the CSF, whether blood, infection, or malignancy, may cause rise in temperature. After subarachnoid haemorrhage, there may also be hypothalamic effects from vasospasm.

Korsakoff's psychosis occurs presumably from ischaemia affecting the limbic system in the temporal lobes. (See Q.180)

135. A C D

Butyrophenones such as haloperidol are perhaps even more prone than the phenothiazines such as perphenazine to produce extrapyramidal side effects. These include, in addition to parkinsonism, acute dystonia, akathisia (restlessness) and tardive dyskinesia. (See Q.14 Page 139)

136. B D E

Sensory loss — and especially loss of joint position sense — allows potential for joint damage. Neuropathic (Charcot) joints also occur in tabes dorsalis, congenital insensitivity to pain and in any severe sensory neuropathy.

137. Primary open-angle (simple) glaucoma

A characteristically gives rise to signs before symptoms
B is a familial disorder
C may present as an acute painful red eye
D gives characteristic visual field defects
E is usually treated initially by surgery

138. Anterior uveitis is the most characteristic ocular manifestation of

A rheumatoid arthritis
B cranial arteritis
C systemic lupus erythematosus
D Behcet's disease
E ankylosing spondylitis

139. Retinal exudates are a characteristic finding in

A Marfan's syndrome
B tabes dorsalis
C retinal vein thrombosis
D amyloidosis
E Gaucher's disease

140. Ocular signs or symptoms are recognised features of

A sarcoidosis
B rosacea
C perioral dermatitis
D lichen planus
E acne vulgaris

Answers overleaf

137. A B D

By far the commonest variety of primary glaucoma, this disease is one of insidious onset and progression. There are arcuate scotomata, peripheral field loss, and excavated pale optic discs. Central vision is preserved until late, which tends to delay presentation. Treatment is essentially medical and based on parasympathomimetic and beta blocker eyedrops. Carbonic anhydrase inhibitor drugs are also used.

138. D E

Keratoconjunctivitis sicca is common and episcleritis and scleritis are important manifestations of rheumatoid disease. Cranial arteritis may lead to ischaemia of the optic nerve and blindness. Although SLE can produce inflammatory changes anywhere in the eye, the most frequent sign of ocular involvement is retinal exudates (colloid bodies). Recurrent anterior uveitis is the most commonly disabling complication of Behcet's disease. (See Q.101 and Q.223)

139. C

The major eye condition in Marfan's syndrome is dislocation of the lens. Severe myopia, glaucoma and retinal detachment occur. The characteristic eye manifestation of tabes in addition to the Argyll-Robertson pupil is primary optic atrophy.

140. A B

In sarcoidosis ocular complications are recognised in 10-25% of cases. Usually, the lesion is uveitis, acute or chronic, but occasionally retino-choroiditis, kerato-conjunctivitis sicca, calcium deposits, ophthalmoplegia and optic nerve lesions are found. In rosacea, about 50% of patients have eye complications such as conjunctivitis, blepharitis, chalazion, keratitis or hordeolum of which keratitis is the most important.

141. Tinea capitis

A is most commonly caused by the fungus *Microsporum*
B is a frequent manifestation of immunological deficiency
C results in permanent alopecia
D can be diagnosed by fluorescence under Wood's light
E is effectively treated with nystatin cream

142. Features of hyaline membrane disease of the newborn include

A chest wall recession
B decreased lung compliance
C increased lung surfactant
D hyperpyrexia
E liability to chest infections in later childhood

143. In athetosis

A cerebral anoxia at birth is a common cause
B a majority of patients have epileptic fits
C over 50% of patients are of severely subnormal intelligence
D the diagnosis if frequently not apparent until after 6 months of age
E deafness is more common than in other types of cerebral palsy

144. Convulsions in the first week of life are a characteristic of

A hypocalcaemia
B postmaturity
C craniopharyngioma
D Werdnig-Hoffman disease
E hypomagnesaemia

Answers overleaf

141. A D

Microsporum species are the commonest causes of tinea of the scalp. *Trichophyton* is an occasional cause. Immunological deficiency may underlie *Candida albicans* infections, but not especially infection with the ringworm fungi. The alopecia caused by the infection should clear up completely with effective treatment. Nystatin is an effective drug only in candidiasis and is ineffective in any form of ringworm. The fluorescence under the ultraviolet rays arising from a Wood's light gives a quick and reliable method of diagnosis. Culture of the fungus is possible, though slow.

142. A B

Lung compliance, i.e. the ability of the lung to expand and collapse in response to pressure changes is markedly reduced in hyaline membrane disease, and this is associated with decreased lung surfactant. The temperature is often subnormal. After recovery the lungs are normal in structure and function, and there is no increase in susceptibility to infections later.

143. A D E

Nearly all cases of athetosis have a clearcut cause of which cerebral anoxia at birth is the commonest nowadays. Fits occur only in a small minority of athetoids but more commonly in spastics. The intellectual level, however, is generally higher in athetoids than in spastics.

Although there may be clues to the diagnosis of athetosis in the early months e.g. a persistent asymmetrical tonic reflex and hypotonia, it is rarely established with certainty before one year of age.

144. A E

There are no particular neurological sequelae of postmaturity, and no association with neonatal convulsions. Craniopharyngioma does often present with a fit, but virtually never in the newborn period. Werdnig-Hoffman disease is a degeneration of the anterior horn cells and cranial motor nuclei. There is no liability to fit. Fits, however, are recognised sequelae of a low calcium or magnesium in the first week.

145. Breast development in a five year old girl

A may be due to an arrhenoblastoma of the ovary
B frequently has no identifiable organic cause
C is a common result of XXY chromosomal constitution
D requires urgent laparotomy to examine the ovaries
E may be a late result of maternal oestrogens transmitted before birth

146. True precocious puberty in a five year old boy

A is most commonly of constitutional (non-organic) cause
B is a late result of untreated congenital adrenal hyperplasia (adreno-genital syndrome)
C is less common than precocious puberty in girls
D is commonly due to the XYY chromosome constitution
E is a recognised sequel of encephalitis

147. The following conditions are characteristically associated with mental retardation:

A osteogenesis imperfecta tarda
B histidinaemia
C Klinefelter's syndrome
D maple-syrup urine disease
E Fanconi syndrome

148. Idiopathic hypercalcaemia in the first year of life

A may result from a renal tubular reabsorption defect
B has an association with aortic stenosis
C frequently presents with convulsions
D may give rise to permanent mental retardation
E causes the radiological changes of rickets

Answers overleaf

145. B

Arrhenoblastoma of the ovary is a very rare tumour, almost confined to adults, and causes androgen (not oestrogen) secretion. Breast development is frequently the first manifestation of constitutional precocious puberty in a girl, with no recognisable organic changes. (It follows, therefore, that laparotomy to examine the ovaries is rarely necessary.) The XXY chromosome constitution (Klinefelter's syndrome) results in a phenotypic male and gynaecomastia occurs at or after the usual time of puberty. Maternal oestrogens frequently cause breast enlargement in newborn babies, both male and female, but it dies away within 2-3 weeks of birth.

146. C E

In contrast to the situation in girls, true precocious puberty in boys is almost always due to organic intracranial lesions, or the effects of previous cerebral disease such as encephalitis. Congenital adrenal hyperplasia, if untreated, would give rise only to the secondary sex characteristics, but not true puberty (i.e. the testes would not enlarge and give rise to spermatogenesis, but would actually atrophy See Q.153). Precocious puberty is very much more common in girls than boys. The XYY constitution may cause no physical effects or may be associated with tall stature, acne, and personality disorder. It does not cause precocious puberty.

147. C D

Individuals with the mild variant of osteogenesis have an increased tendency to fractures, and otosclerosis, but there is no intellectual retardation. Patients with the Fanconi syndrome have severe metabolic effects involving the liver, skeleton etc., but are not mentally retarded. With histidinaemia the picture is less clear-cut but the prevailing view now is that whilst most patients show speech retardation, only a few individuals show true mental retardation. In this respect it is unusual among inborn errors of metabolism.

148. B D

A renal tubular leak of phosphate will result in a low blood phosphate level and probably rickets, but there is no increase in blood calcium. The association of aortic stenosis with severe idiopathic hypercalcaemia has been well described, and is probably due to distortion of the valve by calcium deposition. Mental retardation is an early feature, but convulsions do not occur. The radiological changes include dense metaphyseal plates, denseness of the base of the skull and orbital margins and the "bone-within-a-bone" effect in vertebral bodies, but not rickets.

149. If a child in a children's ward develops measles, the following action is appropriate:

A close the ward to all admission for two weeks
B actively immunise all the other patients against measles
C give gamma globulin to all patients who have not been immunised or had measles
D forbid visiting by the parents until the rash has gone
E give prophylactic antibiotics to all contacts at home

150. At the age of eight months, a baby can be expected to

A roll over from front to back
B pick up a small bead between thumb and finger
C sit up with a straight back
D say up to five words clearly
E feed himself with a spoon

151. In spastic diplegia

A about 75% of patients are of severely subnormal intelligence
B about 30% of patients suffer from epilepsy
C dislocation of the hips commonly occurs in the early years of life
D the diagnosis is usually apparent in the first month of life
E there is strong familial tendency

152. In Down's syndrome

A the commonest congenital heart lesion is patent ductus arteriosus
B there is an increased incidence of acute lymphocytic leukaemia
C cases due to translocation are associated with increased maternal age
D foetal blood sampling should be offered to all pregnant women over the age of 36 years
E borderline clinical features suggest mosaicism

Answers overleaf

149. C

Closure of the whole ward is too drastic a measure following the occurrence of a single case. Active immunisation would take too long to produce the necessary immunity and would not prevent the occurrence of secondary cases. In any case, some children will already have had measles or been immunised previously, and for those who have not, passive immunisation with gamma globulin is probably effective. It is quite unnecessary, and harsh, to forbid parents to visit, and of course, prophylactic antibiotics have no place in the prevention of a viral illness.

150. A C

Rolling over (the denotative righting reaction) is acquired by most babies at five months of age, but the ability to pick up a bead between finger and thumb not until about one year. Babies sit up unsupported at eight months and usually feed themselves with a spoon after one year. Most babies say their first words clearly around 12-14 months, but five words will often not be clearly spoken until 14-16 months.

151. B C

Usually about 30% of children with spastic diplegia are of severely subnormal intelligence and the same percentage have epilepsy. Dislocation of the hips commonly occurs in the early years if the adductor spasm of the thighs is very marked. The diagnosis is often not clear until several months have elapsed, and is rarely obvious in the first month. It is very rare to find more than one spastic child in a family (though there is a rare inherited form of spastic paraplegia).

152. B E

The commonest cardiac anomalies are septal defects and valvular stenosis. Cases due to translocation may occur equally at any age of either parent, and indeed in practice are more commonly seen in young parents, since more children are born to younger than older parents.

There is good reason for offering routine amniocentesis to all older mothers (perhaps 36 and over) but foetal blood sampling is not a procedure available to obstetricians in the present state of our knowledge or technique. Mosaicism for the trisomy seems to occur quite frequently, and does indeed show variable features of the syndrome, making diagnosis difficult.

153. In congenital adrenal hyperplasia

A a male infant appears normal at birth
B testicular hypertrophy occurs
C a female infant typically has clitoral hypertrophy and fusion of labia minora
D the presentation may be with saline depletion and shock in the early weeks of life
E ACTH is effective treatment

154. In kwashiorkor

A hypothermia is a recognised complication
B measles is a recognised precipitant
C oedema is mainly due to a protein-losing enteropathy
D the incidence is highest in the first year of life
E the birth of a second child to the mother may be a contributary factor

155. Juvenile chronic arthritis (Still's disease) is typically associated with

A maculo-papular rash
B negative rheumatoid factor
C involvement of the cervical spine
D sacro-iliitis
E involvement of the distal interphalangeal joints

156. Folate deficiency in childhood occurs as a consequence of

A prematurity
B chronic infection
C renal tubular acidosis
D small bowel malabsorption
E haemolysis

Answers overleaf

153. A C D

Male infants with this condition may show slight penile enlargement and pigmentation, but both are very easily overlooked and passed as normal. The testicles are normal in size and will slowly atrophy if the condition is untreated due to the circulating androgens. (See Q.146) The salt-losing syndrome occurs in about 50% of infants with the 21-hydroxylase block variety. ACTH is, of course, ineffective in treatment (and harmful) since the primary defect is of an enzyme required to elaborate cortisol. It is necessary, therefore, to give cortisol in some form to these patients.

154. A B E

Hypothermia may occur in the later stages of the illness when the patient is very weak and lacking in vitality and mobility. Many infectious fevers, including measles, cause severe illness in these patients, and thus bring kwashiorkor to light. Oedema is indeed associated with a low serum albumen, but this is due to dietary deficiency. Whilst it may begin in the first year, it is most commonly seen in tropical areas in the second and third years, after infants are weaned from the breast. Thus the arrival of a second child may be a contributary factor by causing the cessation of lactation when pregnancy occurs.

155. A B C E

Juvenile chronic arthritis (JCA) is a term used to cover a number of conditions. These include adult-type RA (rheumatoid arthritis — with positive rheumatoid factor tests) and Still's disease, a term that has confused by being used also for all patients with JCA. Some patients with Still's do not have much systemic disease (polyarticular), and others have only the odd joint involved (pauciarticular). Ankylosing spondylitis also presents in childhood as JCA, and has a high incidence of HLA — B27 not found in the other subgroups. Still's disease can, rarely, present in adults.

156. A B D E

Folate deficiency typically occurs following a rapid increase in demand for folate and this occurs with massive increases in erythropoiesis and red cell turn-over. The premature infant is folate deficient because insufficient has been transferred across the placenta from the mother — most of the transfer usually taking place in the last trimester. With long-standing infection in childhood, there is often an increased demand for folate and as folate is absorbed throughout the small bowel, it is likely to become deficient in malabsorption.

157. The following mechanisms are involved in the production of the fluid exudate in acute inflammation:

A increased capillary blood pressure
B increased vascular permeability to protein
C breakdown of large molecular tissue proteins
D diapedesis
E chemotaxis

158. The following conditions typically cause central zonal necrosis of the liver:

A yellow fever
B congestive cardiac failure
C phosphorus poisoning
D eclampsia
E carbon tetrachloride

159. The following are characteristic features of malignant tumours:

A abnormal mitoses
B anaplasia
C reactive hyperplasia in the regional lymph nodes
D increased fibrous stroma
E invasiveness

160. In the tuberculous lesion

A initially infiltration with lymphocytes occurs
B there is progressive destruction of the organisms by macrophages
C caseation consists of dead polymorphs
D the presence of numerous giant cells is evidence of healing
E the presence of caseation, macrophages and epithelioid cells is diagnostic

Answers overleaf

157. A B C

Diapedesis is the passive movement of red cells out of vessels, and chemotaxis the directional movement of an organism in response to a chemical stimulus. Both may occur in acute inflammation, but do not contribute to the fluid exudate.

158. B E

Phosphorus poisoning and eclampsia characteristically cause peripheral zonal necrosis. Yellow fever, on the other hand, gives mid-zonal necrosis. The Budd-Chiari syndrome (hepatic vein occlusion) is typically responsible for severe centrilobular necrosis.

159. A B E

In malignancy, mitoses tend to be not only abnormal, but numerous. Anaplasia is used to denote lack of resemblance of a malignant tumour to its parent organ. Invasiveness is the hallmark of malignancy. Some malignant tumours produce a marked fibrous reaction (e.g. scirrhous carcinoma of the breast), but this is exceptional.

160. B

There is initial transient acute inflammation with polymorphs. Caseation consists of altered macrophages and dead tissue cells. Fibroblasts, not giant cells, provide evidence of healing. Although the combination of caseation, macrophages and epithelioid cells is very suggestive of tuberculosis, it is not diagnostic. (See Q.198)

161. On day 7 of the menstrual cycle as compared with day 21, there is

A a lower progesterone concentration
B a lower body temperature
C more developing follicles
D a thicker endometrium
E a fern-like pattern from a smear of cervical mucus

162. The rate of aldosterone secretion

A is controlled by the renin-angiotensin system
B is increased by increased sodium concentrations in the extracellular fluid
C increases when plasma potassium concentrations rise
D is inversely related to plasma volume
E is increased by stimulation of the sympathetic supply to the adrenal gland

163. Cholecystokinin-pancreozymin (CCK-PZ)

A is released from cells in the pancreatic ducts
B is secreted in response to large amounts of circulating fatty acids
C causes relaxation of the sphincter of Oddi
D causes contraction of the gall bladder
E acts synergistically with secretin

164. Systemic blood pressure is increased

A on the assumption of the upright from the supine position
B on sudden exposure to cold
C always when heart rate increases
D by brain stem asphyxia
E in response to stimulation of peripheral chemoreceptors

Answers overleaf

161. A B C E

The first phase of the menstrual cycle, the follicular phase, is characterised by the development of the follicles. The progesterone concentrations and hence, the body temperature, is lower than in the luteal phase of the cycle. Proliferation of the endomentrium occurs in the second half of the cycle, and so the endometrium is relatively thinner on day 7. A cervical smear on day 7 gives a characteristic fern-like appearance.

162. A C D

Aldosterone sercretion is largely controlled via the renin-angiotensin system, and is inversely related to plasma volume. Plasma potassium concentrations also influence aldosterone release. Aldosterone secretion is greater when the subject is on a low sodium diet. It is the adrenal medulla, not the cortex, which is controlled by the sympathetic nervous system.

163. C D E

CCK-PZ is produced by the intestinal mucosa. It is released following the ingestion of fat in a meal, but not necessarily by large amounts of circulating fatty acids. It aids in the digestion of fats by causing contraction of the gall bladder and relaxation of the sphincter of Oddi. It acts synergistically with secretin in the control of pancreatic secretion.

164. B D E

Blood pressure may be given by the following equation;

$$\text{Blood Pressure} = \text{Cardiac Output} \times \text{Peripheral Resistance.}$$

Therefore, it rises when peripheral resistance increases on exposure to cold. It falls when venous return and hence cardiac output falls. It does not necessarily increase when the heart rate increases, as an increase in heart rate does not necessarily produce an increase in cardiac output. Stimulation of the peripheral chemoreceptors and hypoxia itself act on the pressor area in the medulla to give an increase in blood pressure.

165. Renal blood flow

A is $\frac{1}{5}$-$\frac{1}{4}$ of the total cardiac output
B falls with exercise
C is increased by sympathetic nervous system overactivity
D rises with anaemia
E is constant over the range of mean blood pressure 90-200 mm Hg

166. Airways resistance

A comes largely from the small peripheral airways
B increases in response to increased sympathetic activity
C increases in response to increased parasympathetic activity
D is greater in inspiration than expiration
E is increased in response to stimulation of the pulmonary stretch receptors

167. Vasopressin (ADH)

A is synthesised in the hypothalamus
B is a steroid
C increases permeability of the loop of Henle to water
D is released in response to a fall in blood volume
E relaxes smooth muscle

168. The gastro-oesophageal junction in man

A constitutes an anatomical sphincter
B shows a pressure rise above resting values after completion of the act of swallowing
C relaxes under the influence of gastrin
D has a lower resting pressure in subjects with a sliding hiatus hernia
E shows a rise in pressure after adminstration of metoclopramide

Answers overleaf

165. A B E

Renal blood flow is reduced in exercise when large amounts of blood pass to the muscles. Stimulation of the renal nerves causes vasoconstriction. In contrast to most tissues, renal blood flow tends to fall with anaemia and rises with polycythaemia thus keeping plasma flow constant. Blood transfusion in chronic renal failure can sometimes lead to a serious fall in renal plasma flow. Autoregulation occurs in the kidney so that the blood flow remains constant over the range of blood pressures 90-200 mm Hg.

166. A C

Airways resistance is the pressure difference required per unit of air flow and depends largely on the small peripheral airways, because of their small diameter and large overall cross-sectional area. Increased sympathetic activity dilates the bronchi, while parasympathetic activity constricts them. The resistance is greater on expiration, not inspiration, hence *expiratory* wheezes in asthma.

167. A D

ADH is a nonapeptide believed to be synthesised in the supraoptic and paraventricular nuclei of the hypothalamus and transported along nerve axons to the posterior hypothalamus. It increases the permeability to water of the renal collecting ducts (both cortical and medullary). The osmolar gradients mean that water leaves the tubule thus concentrating the urine. ADH release by falls in blood volume (real or "apparent") may over-ride osmotic changes tending to inhibit release. In large concentrations (e.g. when used therapeutically) vasopressin causes smooth muscle contraction.

168. B E

The gastro-oesophageal junction in man has the characteristics of a physiological sphincter in that it is a zone of relatively high pressure which relaxes its tone prior to the arrival of the oesophageal peristaltic wave and then assumes a higher pressure after its passage before returning to its resting value. Although in other mammals anatomical features of a sphincter are seen, these have not been demonstrated in man. Drugs and hormones have a selective action, gastrin increasing the tone as does metoclopramide, making it a useful drug in the prevention of reflux. Resting pressures in normal subjects and those with hiatus hernia are similar. It is the displacement of the gastro-oesophageal junction above the diaphragm that makes reflux more likely to occur.

169. Typical features of dementia include

A selective impairment of recall
B perseveration of themes
C generalised cortical atrophy
D disorientation in place
E depression

170. The following statements regarding compensation neurosis are correct:

A it has a recognised association with major rather than minor accidents
B it occurs particularly after head injuries sustained at work
C it commonly clears up after settlement of the compensation claim
D malingering accounts for at least 30% of cases
E irritability is a recognised feature

171. Grief reaction

A is typically self-limiting
B characteristically includes denial
C is best treated with tricyclic antidepressants
D typically includes suicidal ideas
E is a form of psychosis

172. Typical features of alcohol withdrawal include

A dehydration
B visual hallucinations
C passivity feelings
D tremor
E confabulation

Answers overleaf

169. A B C D E

In dementia, there is a selective impairment of memory for recent events in the early stages. Later, this generalises and eventually extends to loss of memory for distant events too. There is difficulty in adapting to new situations, so the patient persists or perseverates with old themes. The memory loss is accompanied by disorientation, which may be in time, place, or person. Depression is quite common in early dementia. The dementing process is a result of slowly progressive cortical disease resulting in cortical atrophy.

170. B C E

The incidence of compensation neurosis has an inverse relationship with the severity of the injury. It is twice as common after industrial injuries as after road traffic accidents. The vast majority of patients will be fit to return to work after settlement of the claim, which usually takes about two years. The main symptoms are headaches, dizziness, poor concentration and irritability. Malingering is not a common occurrence, and the mechanisms involved in producing these symptoms are subconscious ones.

171. A B D

The initial stage of a grief reaction is a period of numbness with little or no emotional reaction. This is the period of denial. Subsequent stages follow to a state of depression, and suicidal ideas are often expressed. These may reflect feelings of guilt or identification with the dead person. The reaction is self-limiting although there may be delays up to several years. The treatment of choice would be some form of psychotherapy or counselling. The reaction is neurotic rather than psychotic.

172. A B D

Delirium tremens on withdrawal from alcohol includes a coarse, persistent tremor of the hands. Often, the patient experiences visual hallucinations such as seeing animals crawling on the floor or the bedclothes. There is free perspiration, oliguria and dehydration. Passivity feelings are features of schizophrenia. Confabulation, part of Korsakoff's syndrome, is a result of chronic alcohol abuse, not of acute withdrawal. (See Q.130, Q.134 and Q.180)

173. Good prognostic signs in schizophrenia include

A early onset
B depressive features
C echolalia
D preservation of affect
E visual hallucinations

174. The following information may reasonably be given to patients starting a course of tricyclic antidepressants:

A they should expect the drug to take effect within 24 hours
B they should avoid cheese
C they may experience a dry mouth at first
D their skin may become sensitive to sunlight
E it may help them to lose weight

175. Factors indicating an increased risk of suicide in a depressed patient include

A family history of suicide
B insomnia
C pressure of serious physical illness
D living alone
E presence of paranoid delusions

176. Agoraphobia

A usually starts before puberty
B occurs more often in women than men
C can be effectively treated by systematic desensitisation
D becomes worse during periods of depression
E can usually be traced back to traumatic events in childhood

Answers overleaf

173. B D

The patient with early onset schizophrenia usually suffers more chronic personality deterioration. The presence of affective change, depression or mania seems to indicate preservation of personality and a better prognosis. There is no evidence that any individual symptom such as visual, rather than auditory, hallucinations influences prognosis. Echolalia is usually a symptom of organic brain damage.

174. C

Tricyclic anti-depressants take at least ten days to have their effect. They have no interaction with food as do the monoamineoxidase inhibitors, and do not induce sensitivity to sunlight as do the phenothiazines. They have no direct affect on weight, except that as the depression resolves, the appetite should improve. Initial side effects include dry mouth, but this usually clears up after a few days. Patients should be given this information so that they are encouraged to persist with treatment.

175. A B C D

Symptomatically, depressed suicides resemble an unselected sample of depressives, but they score higher on severity of symptoms, especially insomnia. Of the social factors, positive family history of suicide, prolonged physical illness and living alone indicate a higher risk. Paranoid delusions can occur in depressive illness, but do not have any special significance in assessing suicide risk.

176. B C D

Agoraphobia generally commences suddenly in adult life following a recent traumatic event. There is a large preponderance of women patients, and a worsening of symptoms can occur as a result of other emotional changes such as a period of depression. Treatment is very difficult, but the condition can respond to desensitisation by systematically introducing the patient to the feared situation.

177. The following are characteristic features of hypomania:

A flight of ideas
B thought insertion
C sexual promiscuity
D delusions of bodily illness
E sleep disturbance

178. Puerperal psychosis

A usually begins within the first three months after childbirth
B is commonly accompanied by clouding of consciousness
C has a favourable prognosis
D characteristically includes auditory hallucinations
E characteristically includes obsessional ruminations

179. Anorexia nervosa

A occurs exclusively in females
B tends to be accompanied by episodes of over-eating
C is characterised by apathy and lassitude
D gives hypokalaemia
E is a cause of primary amenorrhoea

180. Korsakoff's syndrome is

A a recognised complication of alcoholism
B due to vitamin B_{12} deficiency
C characterised by generalised deterioration of intellect
D characterised by recent memory defect
E associated with nystagmus

Answers overleaf

177. A C E

Flight of ideas, where there is an excessively fluent flow of thoughts and ideas, but with some thread of connection between them, is characteristic of hypomania. Thought insertion is a first rank symptom of schizophrenia. Overactivity and a sense of grandiosity can lead to sexually promiscuous behaviour. Delusions of bodily illness are a feature of depression, not mania. The manic patient is so active he tends to have very little sleep and can become ill through exhaustion.

178. A B C D

By definition, puerperal psychosis begins within the first three months after childbirth. The illness usually starts with a period of delirium. The outlook is favourable. Auditory hallucinations are frequently experienced, but obsessional ruminations are not part of the clinical picture.

179. B D E

The anorectic patient is typically alert and active inspite of severe emaciation. There may be episodes of hyperactivity. Nonetheless, there is a high incidence of depression and, terminally, weakness and apathy predominate. Hypokalaemia is commonly found, often due to self-induced vomiting or purgation. Amenorrhoea, primary and secondary, is a characteristic feature, and may occur before significant weight loss. The typical endocrine findings are low FSH, LH and oestrogen levels; evidence suggests that the fault lies in hypothalamic control of the anterior pituitary.

180. A D E

Korsakoff's syndrome is characterised by a severe memory defect both retrograde and antegrade, i.e. an inability to retain new information. Other mental functions may be more or less intact. Confabulation is common, but not invariable. With Korsakoff's syndrome in chronic alcoholism, beri-beri and prolonged vomiting, Wernicke's encephalopathy is frequently associated, giving nystagmus, ocular palsies and ataxia. Vitamin B_1 deficiency is the major aetiological factor. Korsakoff's syndrome also occurs after head injuries and cerebral anoxia and with cerebral tumours.
(See Q.134 and Q.172)

RENAL DISEASE

181. An increase in the ratio of plasma urea to creatinine is found in patients

A on corticosteriod therapy
B with severe liver disease
C with intestinal haemorrhage
D with uretero-colic anastomosis
E with pyloric stenosis

182. Rapidly progressive glomerulonephritis

A is a recognised complication of sub-acute infective endocarditis
B characteristically gives severe hypertension
C typically presents with overt nephrotic syndrome
D is a recognised association of post-streptococcal glomerulonephritis
E has a poor prognosis

183. Acute renal failure is a recognised complication of

A penicillin therapy
B water intoxication
C Henoch-Schönlein purpura
D paracetamol intoxication
E polymyalgia rheumatica

184. A low level of serum complement (C_3) is a characteristic finding in

A minimal change glomerulonephritis
B mesangio-capillary (membrano-proliferative) glomerulonephritis
C sub-acute infective endocarditis nephritis
D interstitial nephritis
E acute post-streptococcal glomerulonephritis

Answers overleaf

181. A C D E

In addition to glomerular filtration, the major determinant of plasma creatinine concentration is the rate of production which depends on skeletal muscle mass. Urea production, however rapidly rises in catabolic states (with injury, heart failure, infection and corticosteroid therapy) and with increased gastrointestinal absorption of nitrogen (GI haemorrhage, uretero-colic anastomosis, and high protein diet). Urea production falls in severe liver disease. Urea excretion falls in dehydration due to increased renal tubular reabsorption, hence increasing the plasma urea/creatinine ratio. (See Q.192)

182. A D E

The characteristic histological picture is one of extensive glomerular epithelial proliferation, hence the synonym "crescentic glomerulonephritis". The major clinical feature is uraemia developing over weeks or months. The blood pressure is surprisingly normal or only modestly raised. The condition may be idiopathic or occur in association with infection or systemic diseases such as SLE, Henoch-Schönlein purpura, Goodpasture's syndrome or a vasculitic disorder. (See Q.185)

183. A C D

Various penicillins, especially methicillin, are known to give an acute interstitial nephritis. Glomerulonephritis associated with systemic disorders, with infectious diseases, or idiopathic, can lead to acute renal failure. The histology in such cases often shows crescentic glomerulonephritis (See Q.182). Paracetamol poisoning gives acute tubular necrosis and/or the renal failure that occurs in advanced liver failure. (See Q.233) Cranial arteritis, with which polymyalgia may be associated, can rarely involve the aorta and lead to aneurysm or dissection.

184. B C E

A low serum complement level is also found with glomerulonephritis with SLE and infected ventriculoatrial shunts. One variety of mesangio-capillary glomerulonephritis is characterised by the presence of a protein in the serum (C_3 nephritic factor) that can induce C_3 cleavage in vitro.

185. The following statements about Goodpasture's syndrome are correct:

A the lung lesions are typically cavitating
B the serum complement level is generally normal
C renal biopsy reveals immunofluorescent evidence of anti-glomerular basement membrane antibody
D plasma exchange is of proven therapeutic value
E the typical patient is elderly and female

186. In a patient found to be severely uraemic, the following would indicate chronic renal disease:

A heavy proteinuria
B hyperkalaemia
C skin pigmentation
D urinary osmolality 300 m osmol/kg
E hyponatraemia

187. Typical features of acute post-streptococcal glomerulonephritis include

A a history of previous attacks
B papilloedema
C complete anuria
D a sore throat 10 days previously
E a nephrotic syndrome

188. The following are typical associations of polycystic disease of the kidneys in adults:

A subarachnoid haemorrhage
B nephrolithiasis
C polycythaemia
D liver failure
E nephrotic syndrome

Answers overleaf

185. B C D

The typical patient is a young male adult, but the condition can occur at any age. The first symptoms are usually due to lung haemorrhage. (See Q.204) Sometimes the patient presents with glomerulonephritis, which develops in all patients, and is usually severe. (See Q.182) Plasma exchange in combination with cytotoxic drugs and corticosteroids is proving invaluable therapeutically if there is residual renal function.

186. C

It can sometimes be difficult to distinguish acute renal failure and an acute presentation of end-stage renal disease, although a full history often provides the necessary clues. Other evidence that one is dealing with longstanding renal failure is the presence of renal osteodystrophy, uraemic neuropathy or small kidneys.

187. D

There is good immunity to an infection with nephritogenic Group A beta-haemolytic streptococci, identifiable by the presence of a specific cell-wall antigen (M-protein). A second attack is thus extremely unusual. Severe hypertension with papilloedema, complete anuria and a nephrotic syndrome all occur exceptionally in acute post-streptococcal glomerulonephritis, but their presence should raise the strong possibility of one of the many other causes of "acute nephritis".

188. A B C

Berry aneurysms and urinary stones occur in about 10% of cases. Although liver cysts are found in perhaps a third of cases, they rarely give rise to symptoms and probably never to liver failure. This is in contrast to the much rarer polycystic disease of childhood, where liver failure and portal hypertension due to hepatic fibrosis may be the dominant clinical features.

189. Recurrent haematuria is a recognised feature of

A sickle cell disease
B diabetes mellitus
C acute intermittent porphyria
D proliferative glomerulonephritis
E haemophilia

190. Ureteric obstruction is a characteristic complication of

A membranous glomerulonephritis
B analgesic nephropathy
C schistosomiasis
D renal transplantation
E renal amyloidosis

191. In classical (distal type 1) renal tubular acidosis (RTA) in adults, the following are characteristic findings:

A polyuria
B aminoaciduria
C hyperchloraemia
D uraemia
E ureteric colic

192. The following factors in a patient with acute renal failure would favour the use of peritoneal dialysis (PD) rather than haemodialysis

A myocardial infarction
B chronic bronchitis
C advanced age
D hypotension
E hypercatabolic renal failure

Answers overleaf

189. A D E

Sickle cell disease can produce severe and disabling recurrent bleeding from multiple small renal infarcts especially in the papillae.
Recurrent haematuria, often associated with intercurrent upper respiratory tract infections or exercise, can occur with all the histological varieties of proliferative glomerulonephritis. It is, however, characteristic in lgA nephropathy (Berger's disease), usually showing focal histological changes and prominent mesangial lgA with less lgG and C_3.

190. B C D

Ureteric obstruction occurs in analgesic nephropathy due to sloughed papillae. In schistosomiasis (due to *S. haematobium*), fibrosis occurs in the bladder and ureters, stones are common, and in Egypt, carcinoma of the bladder develops. Ureteric necrosis, due to disturbance of the vascular supply, is a not uncommon complication of transplantation.

191. A C E

Aminoaciduria is found as an associated proximal tubular defect in proximal (type II) RTA. The polyuria is due to impaired osmotic concentrating ability, in part due to hypokalaemia, which also gives muscle weakness. Nephrocalcinosis and urinary stones form due to hypercalciuria, alkaline urine and a low urinary citrate excretion. They may contribute to glomerular failure in some cases, but uraemia is not a typical early feature. The other major problems arise from osteomalacia.

192. A C D

Haemodialysis throws a more severe haemodynamic strain on patients than PD and should be avoided, generally, when the circulatory state is at particular risk after a myocardial infarct in the elderly and the hypotensive. PD, splinting the diaphragms, can lead to respiratory problems even with 1 litre exchanges. It may also not provide adequate urea clearance to correct the uraemia if urea production is especially high. (See Q.181) The optimal urea clearance with PD is about 25-30 ml/min compared with 100ml/min or more for haemodialysis.

193. The following are recognised associations:

A small left pneumothorax and audible systolic "click"
B acute pancreatitis and adult respiratory distress syndrome
C sarcoidosis and bronchial obstruction
D Dressler's (post-myocardial infarction) syndrome and pleural effusion
E nitrofurantoin and chronic pulmonary fibrosis

194. Cavitating lung lesions are characteristic of

A systemic lupus erythematosus
B squamous cell carcinoma
C Wegener's granulomatosis
D progressive massive fibrosis
E "shock" lung

195. The following statements are correct:

A chemoprophylaxis against TB is advisable in Asian patients with Heaf test positive Grade I & II
B BCG is indicated in patients with Heaf test positive Grade IV
C tuberculin PPD is indicated in patients with Heaf test positive Grade IV
D a negative Heaf test is a recognised finding in miliary TB
E Heaf test is of no value in the diagnosis of sarcoidosis

196. The following are recognised treatments of choice:

A lung lavage in alveolar proteinosis
B oral corticosteroids in symptomatic bronchopulmonary aspergillosis
C prophylactic disodiumcromoglycate in exercise-induced asthma
D ampicillin in ornithosis
E erythromycin in thoracic actinomycosis

Answers overleaf

193. A B C D E

"Crunching sounds" or "systolic clicks" can be heard synchronously with the cardiac cycle at the apex with a small left pneumothorax (with or without mediastinal emphysema). Enzymes released in acute pancreatitis damage, amongst other tissues, the lung surfactant and capillaries. Bronchial obstruction in sarcoidosis can be due to endobronchial disease or external compression by enlarged lymph nodes.

Dressler's syndrome has amongst its other features, fever, pericarditis, pneumonitis and arthralgia. Pulmonary fibrosis is a recognised complication of chronic nitrofurantoin therapy. An acute lung reaction can occur within hours of taking the drug. There are chest X-ray changes and often a blood eosinophilia.

194. B C D

Other causes of cavitating lung lesions include tuberculosis, some pneumonias (See Q.201), fungal infections such as aspergillosis, septic and non-septic pulmonary infarction, rheumatoid nodules, and progressive massive fibrosis in silicosis and coal-miners' pneumoconiosis. (See also Q.222)

195. D

The Heaf test is a modified tuberculin test and is graded 0 (negative) to IV (strongly positive). It is depressed and may be negative in sarcoidosis or miliary tuberculosis. Grade O or I indicates no immunity against tuberculosis and hence BCG is indicated.

Grade III or IV in Asians with no active disease may indicate an 'unstable' TB focus and thus chemoprophylaxis is recommended by some centres.

196. A B C

Lung lavage is the single most useful therapy in alveolar proteinosis.

Symptomatic bronchopulmonary aspergillosis requires steroids in the therapy regimen.

Exercise-induced asthma can be diminished or prevented by preliminary inhalation of cromoglycate.

Tetracycline is the treatment of choice in ornithosis and penicillin or tetracycline in thoracic actinomycosis.

197. Surgical resection of carcinoma of the bronchus is contra-indicated in the presence of the following:

A grossly widened carina on bronchoscopy
B hoarseness with immobile left vocal chord
C clubbing
D recurrent haemoptysis
E raised mobile right hemi-diaphragm

198. The following are typical findings in patients with sarcoidosis:

A blood lymphocytosis
B depressed skin response to *Candida albicans*
C increased number of circulating T-lymphocytes
D impaired B-lymphocyte function
E epitheloid cell nodules with central necrosis

199. The following statements about hypertrophic osteoarthropathy are correct:

A oat cell carcinoma of the bronchus is the commonest cause
B the arthropathy is typically symmetrical
C the joint pain is relieved by vagotomy below the origin of the recurrent laryngeal nerve
D gynaecomastia is a recognised association
E pretibial myxoedema is a recognised association

200. In a child aged 12 years with bronchiectasis, the following findings suggest a possible aetiology:

A history of chronic diarrhoea
B past history of pertussis pneumonia
C dextrocardia
D mitral stenosis
E positive serological tests for syphilis

Answers overleaf

197. A B

Recurrent haemoptysis is an indication for surgical resection of bronchial carcinoma.
Resection is contra-indicated if mediastinal glands are involved and this may be indicated by a wide carina on bronchoscopy, or chord paralysis (due to pressure on the recurrent laryngeal nerve).
Unlike phrenic nerve palsy, the raised hemidiaphragm of a collapsed lung caused by proximal tumour compression is mobile and like clubbing does not contra-indicate resection.

198. B

In sarcoidosis, the total lymphocyte count is usually normal or depressed, although the number of circulating 'T-cells' may be reduced (hence diminished skin response to candida and tuberculin) and the 'B-cell' function appears normal or hyper-reactive.
Histologically, sarcoid is characterised by epitheloid cell nodules, but, unlike TB, there is no central necrosis (caseation). (See Q.160)

199. B C D

Hypertrophic osteoarthropathy is characterised by clubbing, gynaecomastia, sub-periosteal new bone formation and symmetrical arthropathy the pain of the latter being helped by vagotomy below the origin of the recurrent laryngeal nerve.
Squamous cell carcinoma of the bronchus is the commonest cause.
It should be distinguished from "thyroid acropachy" of which pretibial myxoedema forms a part.

200. A B C

Bronchiectasis may be congenital as part of Kartagener's syndrome (bronchiectasis, dextrocardia and absent frontal sinuses), or it may complicate pertussis (whooping cough) pneumonia. It is also often prominent in cystic fibrosis and agammaglobulinaemia, both of which may present with chronic diarrhoea.

201. In the UK, lung abscess typically complicates pneumonia due to

A pneumococcus
B staphylococcus
C psittacosis
D mycoplasma
E klebsiella

202. Asthmatic attacks in susceptible patients are recognised to be precipitated by

A exercise
B crying
C sudden changes in temperature
D ingestion of paracetamol
E respiratory infection with *Mycoplasma pneumoniae*

203. A 50 year old woman with long-standing bronchiectasis develops ankle oedema. The following would support the diagnosis of amyloidosis:

A palpable spleen
B left ventricular hypertrophy
C clubbing of the toes
D raised blood creatinine
E normal serum albumin

204. Haemoptysis is a characteristic of

A byssinosis
B idiopathic pulmonary haemosiderosis
C aspergilloma
D Goodpasture's syndrome
E asbestosis

Answers overleaf

201. B E

Lung abscesses (necrosis of consolidated areas) frequently complicate staphylococcal and klebsiella pneumonia, but the lesions are usually multiple and bilateral with the former, and single and hence confined to one lobe, in the latter. (See Q.194)

202. A B C E

Recognised trigger factors of asthma include exercise, change in temperature, emotional changes including weeping, respiratory tract infections, and ingestion of aspirin but not paracetamol. (Although a drop in FEV_1 has been reported if paracetamol is given to aspirin sensitive patients.)

203. A D

Amyloid complicating bronchiectasis (secondary amyloid) is deposited predominantly in liver, spleen and kidneys and hence can present with splenomegaly, uraemia and nephrotic syndrome (hypo-albuminaemia, proteinuria and oedema).
Heart involvement is rare in secondary amyloidosis and clubbing is a feature of uncomplicated bronchiectasis.

204. B C D

Haemoptysis is an important part of the clinical picture of idiopathic pulmonary haemosiderosis, aspergilloma and Goodpasture's syndrome (pulmonary haemorrhage and glomerulonephritis with anti-basement membrane antibody; See Q.185). It would be atypical in byssinosis, which is due to inhalation of dusts of cotton, flax or hemp, or in asbestosis unless complicated by lung cancer.

205. An arterial pO_2 of approximately 6·5 kPa (50 mm Hg)

A is a typical finding in fibrosing alveolitis
B implies full saturation of haemoglobin with oxygen
C in asthma will only be found with a raised arterial pCO_2
D indicates that oxygen therapy may be dangerous
E is most frequently due to hypoventilation in chronic lung disease

206. The following are typical features of cryptogenic fibrosing alveolitis (diffuse idiopathic interstitial fibrosis):

A recurrent haemoptysis
B stridor
C finger clubbing
D 'honeycomb' lungs radiologically
E circulating rheumatoid factor

207. "Intrinsic" asthma is characterised by

A an onset in adult life
B high circulating IgE levels
C absence of sputum eosinophilia
D family history of allergies
E a good response to cromoglycate ("Intal")

208. Recognised occupational causes of asthma include

A isocyanates
B platinum salts
C soldering flux
D asbestos
E beryllium

Answers overleaf

205. A

The degree of haemoglobin saturation is predicted by the appropriate oxygen-haemoglobin dissociation curve, but at an arterial pO_2 of 6·5kPa it will be well under 100% and nearer 75%. The commonest cause of hypoxaemia in chronic lung disease is ventilation-perfusion inequality. This is the mechanism of the hypoxaemia which is very common in acute asthma with a low or normal arterial pCO_2. Oxygen therapy is only likely to be dangerous if the arterial pCO_2 is raised and the respiratory drive is dependent on hypoxaemia.

206. C D E

The characteristic symptoms and signs are dyspnoea, cyanosis, clubbing and basal crepitations. Honeycombing is a non-specific appearance of many diffuse lung diseases in an advanced stage. Rheumatoid factor is found in an appreciable percentage of cases; frank rheumatoid arthritis sometimes is associated. There is also an association with chronic active hepatitis, Hashimoto's disease and renal tubular acidosis. (See Q.191)

207. A

The majority of cases of asthma presenting over the age of thirty have "intrinsic" asthma, without personal or family history of atopy and with negative skin tests. They may have vasomotor rhinitis and nasal polyps, and like the "extrinsic" cases, blood and sputum eosinophilia. The majority of younger asthmatics have "extrinsic" disease with raised IgE levels, an atopic background and a tendency to hay fever and seasonal asthma. In practice, however, these distinctions may not be so marked in individual patients.

208. A B C

Isocyanates are used in polyurethane foam manufacture and platinum in the electronics and chemical industries. An increasing number of organic dusts are being recognised as causes of occupational asthma. Asbestosis gives diffuse lung fibrosis and berylliosis is a granulomatous disease resembling sarcoidosis.

209. In alpha$_1$-antitrypsin deficiency

A emphysema is usually most marked in the lower lobes
B the mode of inheritance is autosomal dominant
C the onset of pulmonary symptoms typically occurs in childhood
D atopy is a characteristic association
E smoking plays a synergistic role in the development of emphysema

210. Characteristic features of pulmonary hypertension include

A dominant S wave in ECG lead V_1
B large "a" wave in jugular venous pulse
C exertional dyspnoea
D angina
E clubbing

211. Pleural calcification occurs in

A silicosis
B asbestosis
C haemothorax
D tuberculosis
E haemosiderosis

212. A high protein content is characteristic of pleural effusions associated with

A tuberculosis
B cirrhosis
C bronchogenic carcinoma
D congestive heart failure
E rheumatoid disease

Answers overleaf

209. A E

Alpha$_1$-antitrypsin deficiency is associated with severe panacinar emphysema and is an autosomal recessive condition. Patients present in early adult life, usually before the age of 40 and the emphysema is more severe in cigarette smokers. Children with alpha$_1$-antitrypsin deficiency are prone to severe liver disease such as neonatal hepatitis and cirrhosis. (See Q.32 Page 128)

210. B C D

The ECG changes might include right axis deviation, dominant R waves over the right sided praecordial leads and evidence of right atrial hypertrophy (See Q.26). Exertional dyspnoea in pulmonary hypertension without lung disease, or left sided heart disease has been attributed to ischaemia of the muscles of respiration. Finger clubbing is likely if the cause of the pulmonary hypertension is destructive lung disease or cyanotic heart disease, but is not a sign of pulmonary hypertension itself.

211. B C D

Silicosis gives calcification of intra-thoracic lymphglands producing an 'egg-shell' appearance. The extensive pleural plaques of asbestosis with interlobar, diaphragmatic and pericardial location is often diagnostic. Haemosiderosis gives intra-pulmonary calcification.

212. A C E

An approximate dividing line between exudates and transudates is a protein content of 30g/l. Other causes of exudative pleural effusions include bacterial infections, metastatic carcinoma, pulmonary infarction and acute pancreatitis.

213. The following may be manifestations of rheumatoid arthritis:

A erythema multiforme
B erythema nodosum
C pericardial tamponade
D digital gangrene
E amyloidosis

214. Radiological bone erosions are a typical finding in

A hyperparathyroidism
B Wegener's granulomatosis
C gout
D systemic lupus erythematosus
E psoriatic arthritis

215. The following are recognised features of polyarteritis nodosa:

A positive hepatitis B serology
B asthma
C mononeuritis multiplex
D myalgia
E increased incidence in females

216. Carpal tunnel syndrome is

A often bilateral in amyloidosis
B a cause of wasting of abductor pollicis brevis
C diagnosed by finding delayed ulnar nerve conduction
D a possible cause of pain in the forearm
E significantly associated with obesity

Answers overleaf

213. C D E

Rheumatoid pericardial (and pleural) effusions are characterised by low glucose and complement concentrations (See Q.212). Digital gangrene in rheumatoid disease is a manifestation of a vasculitis which also gives nail fold thrombi and leg ulcers.

214. A C E

Gout and psoriatic arthritis can both cause relatively coarse erosion of bone adjacent to affected joints. A finer bony destruction especially subperiosteal is typical of the osteitis fibrosis cystica of hyperparathyroidism. Important sites to examine are the middle phalanges, the symphysis pubis and skull. Erosions have been reported in SLE but are excessively rare and are not typical. Wegener's granulomatosis is typified by necrotising lesions of nasal mucosa, lung, kidney, joints, skin and nervous system. (See Q.194)

215. A B C D

About 20% of patients with polyarteritis carry hepatitis B surface antigen (See Q.71). It may present with vague symptoms of general malaise and weight loss as well as rash including purpura and fever. Late onset asthma may be the only symptom with pulmonary infiltrates and/or eosinophilia, but myalgia, especially calf pain, is a common symptom. Peripheral neuropathy occurs in ½ - ⅔ of cases of which mononeuritis multiplex in turn accounts for half. In contrast with most of the other connective tissue diseases, polyarteritis nodosa is commoner in men.

216. A B D

The common causes of carpal tunnel syndrome are pregnancy, hypothyroidism, acromegaly and rheumatoid arthritis, but a proportion of the last-named cause are due to bilateral amyloid deposits which can be demonstrated histologically after division of the flexor retinaculum. Delayed median nerve conduction is its hallmark and abductor pollicis brevis wasting largely contributes to the thenar eminence wasting. It is difficult to explain how the pain often radiates as proximally as the elbow, but it is a common symptom.

217. The following are features of systemic sclerosis:

A calcinosis
B an association with intra-abdominal malignancy
C myopathy
D central nervous system involvement
E an association with primary biliary cirrhosis

218. Mixed connective tissue disease

A is an "overlap syndrome" of SLE, systemic sclerosis and myositis
B is diagnosed by the presence of anti-ribonucleoprotein antibodies
C typically has raised titres of anti-DNA antibodies
D carries a better prognosis than systemic sclerosis
E typically causes renal impairment

219. Drug-induced systemic lupus erythematosus is

A equally common in men and women
B significantly more common in fast than slow acetylators
C not generally complicated by renal disease
D caused by sulphonamides
E irreversible, even after drug withdrawal

220. Joint pain and swelling is a recognised feature of

A idiopathic thrombocytopenic purpura
B Christmas disease (factor IX deficiency)
C acute post-streptococcal glomerulonephritis
D sarcoidosis
E amyloidosis

Answers overleaf

217. A C E

The CRST syndrome (calcinosis, Raynaud's, sclerodactyly, telangiectasia) is considered a milder variant of systemic sclerosis. Whereas the feature of myopathy runs throughout the spectrum of connective tissue diseases, CNS complications are not a feature of systemic sclerosis and are more characteristic of SLE. However, systemic sclerosis can cause resistant malignant hypertension which could, in turn, cause cerebrovascular disease. Polymyositis and dermatomyositis in adults are associated with underlying malignancy. (See Q.132)

218. A B D

Sharp in 1973 analysed a group of patients with antibodies against "extractable nuclear antigen" (ENA) and found that they had clinical similarities. ENA has since been shown to contain ribonucleoprotein (RNP), the specific antigen. Raynaud's phenomenon is virtually always present. The presence of raised titres of anti-DNA antibody would push the diagnosis to one of SLE. It is thought to have a better prognosis than systemic sclerosis and this is mainly due to the virtual absence of serious renal disease. (See Q.218)

219. A C D

Drug-induced SLE is equally common in men and women whereas "idiopathic" SLE has a 9 : 1 female to male preponderance. The list of drugs that may precipitate lupus includes sulphonamides, isoniazid, griseofulvin, hydralazine, procainamide and carbamazepine. Slow acetylators are more prone and slower metabolism of the drugs is important. Drug-induced SLE is virtually never complicated by renal disease. Withdrawal of the offending drug leads to disappearance of the disease, but complete reversal has been recorded as taking up to 2 years in some cases of hydralazine-induced SLE.

220. B D E

Christmas disease is indistinguishable clinically from haemophilia, and haemarthrosis is a major clinical problem. Arthritis is not a feature of thrombocytopenia, although prominent in Henoch-Schönlein purpura. Arthralgia and arthritis occur in sarcoidosis with erythema nodosum and, more chronically, in more indolent disease. Amyloid arthropathy, which is seen especially in multiple myeloma, can mimic rheumatoid arthritis.

221. The following statements regarding pseudo-gout (chondrocalcinosis) are correct:

A acute arthritis involves the knee more often than other joints
B radiological calcification is seen in the intervertebral discs
C the disease may mimic osteoarthritis of the hands
D there is a recognised association with primary hyperparathyroidism
E colchicine provides effective prophylaxis against acute attacks

222. In a patient suspected of having a connective-tissue disorder, the following findings favour systemic lupus erythematosus:

A joint deformities
B cavitating lung lesion
C peripheral neuropathy
D anti-ribonucleoprotein (RNP) antibodies
E severe Raynaud's phenomenon

223. Patients with HLA-B27 type who have the following diseases are especially liable to develop sacro-iliitis:

A ulcerative colitis
B Crohn's disease
C gout
D ankylosing spondylitis
E Reiter's syndrome

224. Avascular necrosis of bone is a recognised complication of

A systemic lupus erythematosus
B renal transplantation
C sickle cell disease
D congestive cardiac failure
E Cushing's syndrome

Answers overleaf

221. A B C D

Calcium pyrophosphate dihydrate crystais, which are weakly positively birefringent, are deposited in cartilage and can be seen in joint fluid. Chronic forms of the disease without acute attacks may mimic osteoarthritis, chronic gout, or rheumatoid arthritis. There is no effective prophylactic drug for acute attacks, although nonsteroidal anti-inflammatory drugs can be used.

222. None

Joint deformities are uncommon in SLE and their presence would favour rheumatoid arthritis. A lung cavity would suggest Wegener's disease, peripheral neuropathy (especially if mononeuritis multiplex), polyarteritis nodosa, RNP antibodies, mixed connective tissue disease and severe Raynaud's, systemic sclerosis or mixed connective tissue disease. (See Q.194 and Q.128)

223. A B D E

HLA-B27 has a prevalence of about 7% in a Caucasian population and about 90% in patients with ankylosing spondylitis. There is also a high incidence of HLA-B27 in patients with isolated anterior uveitis. (See Q.138)
Patients with psoriasis have a high incidence of certain other HLA antigens. However, there is a high incidence of HLA-B27 in those with associated sacroiliitis and spondylitis and a much lower one in those with peripheral arthritis only.

224. A B C E

The precise aetiology is unknown and cannot be purely a problem of inadequate blood supply. There are many causes including SLE (though treatment by corticosteroids may be contributory), sickle cell disease and Cushing's syndrome (presumably high corticosteroid output). Again the immuno-suppressive treatment including prednisolone given to renal transplant patients is also considered causative.

225. The following statements are correct:

A a histogram is a univariate frequency diagram
B in a normal or Gaussian distribution the mean, mode and median are different
C when a distribution is negatively skewed, the mean will usually be lower than the mode
D when a distribution is negatively skewed, the median will usually be higher than the mode
E the coefficient of variation is derived from the range

226. The following are true of a normal distribution:

A 95% of observations lie within mean $\pm$ 1 standard deviation (SD)
B 2·5% of observations lie below 2 standard deviations of the mean
C Student's t-test could be used to compare the data with those of another population which is normally distributed
D a non parametric test may be used to compare the data with those of another population
E 99% of observations lie within 2·6 standard errors of the mean

227. The following are true for ischaemic heart disease:

A the prevalence reflects the number of new cases reported annually
B the incidence indicates the total number of cases in the population at a given time
C there is a significant association between hypertension and ischaemic heart disease
D it is absolutely certain that cigarette smoking contributes to the development of heart disease
E the true relationship between smoking and ischaemic heart disease may be accurately assessed by simple bivariate correlation analysis

228. The following statements are correct:

A the standard error of the mean (SEM) provides an index of the spread of observations around the mean
B the standard error of the mean is calculated as the square root of the variance
C the standard deviation is generally smaller than the standard error of the mean
D the standard deviation is an index of the reliability of the mean
E one advantage of the standard deviation is that it can be manipulated mathematically

Answers overleaf

225. A C

The mode is the maximum point on a frequency distribution curve i.e. the most frequently observed measurement. The median is the centre value of a series of observations ranged in order of magnitude. In a normal distribution, the mean, mode and median coincide. In a negatively skewed distribution, both the mean and the median are lower than the mode.
The coefficient of variation is a measure of the spread of values irrespective of the units, this is $\frac{\text{standard deviation}}{\text{mean}} \times 100$

The range is the difference between the highest and lowest values and gives no measure of the distribution of the values in between.

226. B C D

About 68% of observations lie within mean $\pm$ standard deviation. (95% and 99.7% within mean $\pm$ 2 SD and 3SD respectively). Non parametric tests are not as powerful as the Student's t-test and, so might be less desirable. Unlike Student's t-test, non parametric tests (e.g. Mann-Whitney 'U' test or Wilcoxon rank sums test) can be used on data which form a skew distribution. 99% of observations lie within 2·6 standard *deviations* of the mean.

227. C

The prevalence of ischaemic heart disease reflects the total number of cases in the population, whereas the incidence indicates the number of new cases reported annually. There is a significant association between ischaemic heart disease and both smoking and hypertension. However, it is not absolutely certain that these associations are genuine — i.e. the results obtained might have occurred by chance on a small number of occasions. Nothing is *absolutely* certain in biology. Since ischaemic heart disease probably has a multifactorial aetiology (e.g. heredity, lipids, smoking, obesity, etc.) the true relationship between smoking and ischaemic heart disease can only be worked out taking all these factors into account. Multivariate (not bivariate) analysis would be used in this situation.

228. E

The standard deviation gives a measure of the spread of observations around the mean whereas the standard error assesses the reliability of the mean. They are related

$$(\text{SEM} = \text{SD} \div \sqrt{n})$$

in such a way that the standard error of the mean is always the smaller. The standard deviation is calculated as the square root of the variance and its advantage over the mean deviation is that it can be manipulated mathematically.

229. In a preliminary trial a new oral hypoglycaemic agent is administered to 12 diabetic patients:

A the effect on blood glucose will almost certainly be identical in diabetics and in normal subjects
B the statistical significance of the fall in blood glucose may be analysed by Student's unpaired t-test
C if this trial was carried out double blind neither the doctor nor the patient would be aware whether the drug or a placebo was being given
D a fall in blood glucose with a probability value $P > 0 \cdot 05$ would indicate a significant effect on the drug
E one in twenty such studies would be expected to show a significant effect of the hypoglycaemic agent on blood glucose by chance alone

230. The correlation coefficient r between two variables is estimated from a sample of pairs of observations. The following statements are correct:

A if $r = 0 \cdot 9$ there is a very good negative correlation between the two variables
B if $r = 0 \cdot 1$ there is unlikely to be a significant relationship between the two variables
C if $r = 0 \cdot 4$, $p < 0 \cdot 05$ then there is a significant correlation present
D r may be positive or negative
E the Pearson correlation test is ideally used on less than 10 pairs of variables

231. The median is used in preference to the arithmetic mean when

A the variance is large
B the sample size is large
C the observations form a very skew distribution
D the data is normally distributed
E observer error is likely to be large

232. The following are often desirable when carrying out a clinical trial of a new drug:

A apparatus with which to make reproducible observations
B use of a double blind cross-over method
C administration of the drug to patients undergoing treatment with other drugs
D the drug should have been tested extensively in animals
E a pilot study

Answers overleaf

229. C E

Diabetics show different responses to sulphonylureas and biguanides from normal subjects, possibly as a result of beta-cell damage. A new antidiabetic agent might thus behave similarly. The significance of a fall in blood glucose following administration of the drug could be assessed by Student's *paired* t-test, the patients pre-drug level being the control value. A significant fall in blood glucose would be indicated by $P < 0{\cdot}05$. 1 in 20 (5%) such studies would be expected to show a significant effect of the drug on blood glucose by chance alone. This follows from the 5% level being taken conventionally as the level at which statistical significance is achieved.

230. B C D

The correlation coefficient r varies between -1 for a perfect negative correlation to $+1$ for a perfect positive correlation. When $r = 0$ there is no evidence of any relationship between the two variables in question. A $P < 0{\cdot}05$ indicates statistical significance, irrespective of the value of r. The Pearson correlation test should normally be used on more than about 15-18 pairs of variables. For correlation of pairs of variables in a smaller number of subjects Kendall or Spearman rank correlation tests could be used.

231. C

The median is used in preference to the arithmetic mean only when the observations form a very skew distribution. In such a situation, two or three very abnormal observations might disturb the role of the arithmetic mean as a measure of central location. The median cannot be mathematically manipulated.

232. A B D E

A number of conditions are desirable when carrying out a clinical trial of a new drug. Firstly, the drug should be safe and have been thoroughly tested in experimental animals. A pilot study is useful to help the design of the proper study, in particular to predict the number of observations required to attain a result of statistical significance. A double blind cross-over method is a well-tried and effective design, but is not uniformly applicable and can give rise to problems in certain circumstances. It is usually best to administer the drug to patients who are not undergoing treatment with other drugs as these may interfere with the results.

TOXICOLOGY

233. Paracetamol poisoning

A is the commonest cause of acute liver failure in the UK
B causes liver damage after conversion by liver enzymes to a toxic metabolite
C will give rise to permanent liver damage if the patient survives an episode of acute hepatic failure
D is treated with acetyl cysteine or methionine to enhance glutathione conjugation
E may cause acute tubular necrosis of the kidney

234. Inorganic arsenic given in the past may contribute to the occurrence of

A pigmentary changes in the skin
B rodent ulcers on the face
C carcinoma of the bronchus
D epilepsy
E eczema

235. Typical findings in nitrazepam (Mogadon) overdose include

A deep coma
B convulsions
C dilated pupils
D cardiac arrhythmias
E hypothermia

236. An adult has taken 50 aspirin tablets; after four hours

A coma is to be expected
B gastric lavage is of no value
C hyperventilation may occur
D peritoneal dialysis could be of value therapeutically
E hypoglycaemia may be present

Answers overleaf

233. A B D E

Since the first two cases were reported in 1966, the mortality has risen to 419 reported cases in 1977. Hepatic necrosis is not related to blood levels of unaltered paracetamol, but is probably caused by the metabolites produced by mixed function oxidase enzymes (cytochrome P450). These metabolites are partly eliminated by conjugation with glutathione which provides the rationale for administering its precursors acetylcysteine and methionine within 10 hours of paracetamol ingestion. Patients who survive acute liver failure usually make a full recovery. Acute tubular necrosis may occur — usually when there is fulminant liver failure. (See Q.183)

234. A C

Inorganic arsenic may result in guttate (raindrop) hyper-pigmentation and is linked with an increased chance of carcinoma of the bronchus. It is related also to basal cell carcinoma (rodent ulcers) on covered areas, but rodent ulcers on the face are largely related to light exposure and their incidence is not increased by the ingestion of arsenic. Epileptics used to be at risk as regards ingestion of arsenic which was added to bromide anti-epileptic medicines, but epilepsy is not provoked by arsenic ingestion.

235. E

Deep coma would be exceptional and the pupils tend to be constricted. Convulsions may occur but only in the withdrawal phase. The absence of cardiac arrhythmias contrasts with tricyclic antidepressant drug poisoning.

236. C D E

Salicylate is secreted into the stomach long after ingestion. A respiratory alkalosis is the commonest metabolic abnormality in adults, but is only transient in children who develop metabolic acidosis more readily. Although peritoneal dialysis removes salicylate effectively, it is not used unless a forced alkaline diuresis is not possible. Salicylates impair carbohydrate metabolism. (See Q.36)

TROPICAL MEDICINE

237. In leprosy

A the lepromatous form is characteristically associated with a negative lepromin test
B large numbers of *Mycobacterium leprae* are present in the lesions of tuberculoid leprosy
C infected nasal secretions are the main source of infection
D *Mycobacterium leprae* are commonly shed from neuropathic ulcers
E therapy should ideally be on a life-long basis in the lepromatous form

238. The following drugs play an important role in the treatment of the condition mentioned:

A diethylcarbamazine (Banocide) in filarial elephantiasis
B piridazole (Ambilhar) in schistosomiasis
C dapsone in tuberculoid leprosy
D pentavalent antimony in kala-azar
E primaquine in acute falciparum malaria

239. Burkitt's lymphoma is

A confined to Africa
B significantly associated with evidence of Epstein-Barr virus (EBV)
C resistant to anti-tumour chemotherapy
D predominantly a disease of children
E similar to Hodgkin's disease histologically

240. The following statements about beri-beri are correct:

A it can be produced by an experimental diet deficient in thiamine
B it is a complication of alcoholism
C the most common presentation is with high-output cardiac failure
D a raised level of red cell transketolase is diagnostic
E riboflavine deficiency contributes to the disease

Answers overleaf

237. A C E

The lepromin test is characteristically positive in tuberculoid leprosy. *Mycobacterium leprae* are characteristically scanty in tuberculoid leprosy except during a reaction. The diagnosis of leprosy can be made by examining nasal secretions and smears taken from skin and ear biopsies. Therapy is frequently from 3 - 5 years or more, and in the lepromatous form ideally, it should be life-long.

238. B C D

Diethylcarbamazine is given for active Bancroftian filariasis with microfilaria in the blood. It has little to offer with established elephantiasis. Primaquine is used to eradicate persistent hepatic organisms after infection with *P. vivax* or *ovale* (See Q.86). Chloroquine is the drug of choice for all types of acute malaria except chloroquine-resistant *P. falciparum,* when quinine is used.

239. B D

Burkitt's lymphoma is very common in certain areas of East Africa but is found worldwide. In Africa it typically presents with tumours of the facial bones. It is a B-cell lymphoma consisting of undifferentiated lymphoid cells and is generally very sensitive to drugs such as cyclophosphamide. The significance of the association with EBV which is more marked in Africa is unknown.

240. A B

Beri-beri is due solely to deficiency of thiamine although the degree of physical activity and carbohydrate ingestion contribute. However, in practice, other B vitamins are often also deficient. It occurs in western countries in alcoholics, hyperemesis gravidarum, and in other disorders of potential malnutrition such as haemo- and peritoneal dialysis. The majority of cases worldwide have features of a peripheral neuropathy. A *low* red cell transketolase level is of value diagnostically.

PRACTICE EXAM

60 Questions — time allowed 2½ hours

1. **The median nerve**

   A supplies the muscles of the hypothenar eminence
   B supplies the abductor pollicis longus
   C typically supplies the 1st and 2nd lumbricals
   D lies deep to the extensor retinaculum at the wrist
   E supplies the palmar aspect of the index finger

2. **A plasma bicarbonate level of 34 mEg/L would be an unexpected finding in a patient with**

   A hypokalaemia
   B vomiting due to pyloric stenosis
   C untreated diabetic ketoacidosis
   D chronic cor pulmonale
   E chronic renal failure

3. **A high plasma inorganic phosphate level is a characteristic finding in**

   A acromegaly
   B the osteodystrophy of chronic renal failure
   C hypoparathyroidism
   D nutritional rickets
   E Paget's disease

4. **A low plasma sodium (as measured by the auto-analyser) may be a consequence of**

   A bronchial carcinoma
   B salt depletion
   C hyperlipidaemia
   D Cushing's syndrome
   E hyperglycaemia

5. In acute massive pulmonary embolism

A clinical evidence of deep venous thrombosis is characteristically present
B pulmonary embolectomy is the treatment of choice
C the arterial pCO2 is characteristically raised
D the chest X-ray shows oligaemia in the lung fields in a majority of cases
E subcutaneous heparin should be started immediately the diagnosis is suspected

6. The following statements are correct:

A complete heart block is associated with a poor prognosis in anterior myocardial infarction
B complete heart block complicating myocardial infarction characteristically resolves if the patient survives
C the A-V node is supplied by the circumflex coronary artery in 90% of patients
D acute mitral regurgitation associated with myocardial infarction can be easily distinguished from rheumatic mitral regurgitation by the site of the murmur
E the commonest cause of chronic complete heart block is ischaemic heart disease

7. A man of 40 has an untreated blood pressure of 230/125 mm Hg and a plasma potassium of 2·7 m mol/l. A diagnosis of primary aldosteronism is suggested by finding

A soft retinal exudates
B plasma sodium 132 m mol/l
C ankle oedema
D a goitre
E a bruit in the loin

8. Isolated calcific aortic stenosis in the elderly

A is rheumatic in origin in the majority of cases
B may present as congestive cardiac failure
C is associated characteristically with a systolic ejection click
D tends to soften and delay the aortic component of the second sound
E is not haemodynamically important in the absence of a thrill

9. A rumbling apical diastolic bruit is a recognised finding in

A systemic arterial hypertension
B thyrotoxicosis
C mitral regurgitation
D complete heartblock
E ventricular septal defect

10. Glyceryl tri-nitrate

A decreases central venous pressure
B increases stroke volume
C increases pulse pressure
D decreases mean arterial pressure
E increases heart rate

11. The following drugs cause the following urinary tract diseases:

A tetracycline and uraemia
B penicillamine and papillary necrosis
C allopurinol and uric acid nephropathy
D gold and glomerulonephritis
E cyclophosphamide and cystitis

12. The following drug combinations are usually undesirable:

A bendrofluazide and guanethidine
B amitriptyline and bethanidine
C probenecid and penicillin
D ephedrine and a monoamine oxidase inhibitor
E ferrous sulphate and tetracycline

13. Morphine

A is mainly excreted unchanged by the kidneys
B produces mydriasis
C decreases intestinal smooth muscle tone
D decreases peripheral venous capacitance
E is antagonised by naloxone

14. In the treatment of thyrotoxicosis

A iodine and potassium perchlorate are used in combination prior to partial thyroidectomy
B radioactive iodine is contraindicated in children because of the risk of subsequent leukaemia
C lymphocytic infiltration of the surgically removed gland correlates with an increased risk of late hypothyroidism
D radioactive iodine therapy of a toxic adenoma is less likely to result in late hypothyroidism than when used in Graves' disease
E latent hypoparathyroidism, with a normal serum calcium, is a common cause of ill-health following partial thyroidectomy

15. A positive family history is a recognised feature of

A angioedema
B herpes zoster
C psoriasis
D systemic lupus erythematosus
E erythema multiforme

16. Exfoliative dermatitis

A may contribute to heart failure
B gives hyperpyrexia
C with pruritus indicates a lymphoma
D can complicate psoriasis
E may be responsible for lymphadenopathy

17. In patients with non-metastatic manifestations of malignancy

A hypercalcaemia may be suppressed by prednisolone
B thyrotoxicosis associated with chorion carcinoma does not show eye signs
C the commonest tumour to cause polycythaemia is hypernephroma
D ectopic ADH (vasopressin) secretion presents with hypokalaemia
E myasthenia responding to neostigmine is found in association with bronchial carcinoma

18. Phenothiazines may cause

A agranulocytosis
B photosensitivity
C increased lacrimation
D priapism
E cholestatic jaundice

19. In primary hyperparathyroidism there is

A an invariable increase in the level of parathyroid hormone in blood
B an increase in tubular reabsorption of calcium in the presence of hypercalciuria
C the possibility of hypocalcaemic tetany in a neonate whose mother has the condition
D a single adenoma in about 40% of cases
E a recognised association with systemic arterial hypertension

20. Chromophobe adenomas of the pituitary gland

A may be associated with excessive secretion of growth hormone
B rarely cause expansion of the pituitary fossa
C rarely give rise to pituitary failure
D are a recognised association in patients with primary hyperparathyroidism due to hyperplasia of the parathyroid glands
E may progress to involve the supraopticohypophyseal tract thereby causing diabetes insipidus

21. Salivary gland enlargement is a recognised finding in

A amyloidosis
B polycythaemia rubra vera
C sarcoidosis
D alcoholism
E lymphoma

22. In a patient with dysphagia, the following features suggest achalasia rather than carcinoma of the oesophagus:

A absence of spontaneous pain
B difficulty in swallowing both liquids and solids from the onset of symptoms
C sudden and progressive difficulty with drinking
D maintenance of nutritional state if food is eaten slowly
E the initial absence of impaction pain

23. Acute pancreatitis is a recognised complication of

A hypoparathyroidism
B gallstones
C haemochromatosis
D ascariasis
E mumps

24. In idiopathic haemochromatosis

A portal hypertension and liver failure occur more commonly than in Laennec's cirrhosis
B a history of high alcohol consumption is usually present
C repeated venesection does not improve the prognosis
D hepatic pain is a recognised feature
E hepatoma is the commonest cause of death in treated patients

25. Gonorrhoea in the male

A has an incubation period of about 14 days
B is more prone to give disseminated disease than in women
C gives acute epididymitis in about half the cases
D can be prevented by the use of a vaccine
E is a recognised cause of adrenal haemorrhage

26. An acute confusional state is

A often responsive to tricyclic antidepressant drug therapy
B a characteristic feature of myxoedema
C characterised by loss of memory for recent events
D typically reversible
E more common with pre-existing brain disease

27. The following are associated with a prolonged bleeding time:

A haemophilia (Factor VIII deficiency)
B Xmas disease (Factor IX deficiency)
C von Willebrand's disease
D polycythaemia rubra vera
E auto-immune haemolytic anaemia

28. In multiple myeloma

A radiotherapy is a useful means of controlling hypercalcaemia
B the prognosis is closely correlated with blood urea concentration
C hyperviscosity is more common in IgA than IgG types
D peripheral neuropathy is a recognised complication
E the serum alkaline phosphatase is characteristically normal

29. The Medical Officer for Environmental Health must be notified following the presumptive diagnosis of

A meningococcal meningitis
B actinomycosis
C aspergillosis
D measles
E food poisoning

30. Legionnaire's disease

A is contagious
B is treated with high dosage erythromycin
C is significantly associated with abnormal liver function tests
D gives diagnostic radiological findings
E is significantly associated with cigarette smoking

31. The following statements about rubella are correct:

A the period of infectivity is from 5 days before until 4 days after the onset of the rash
B the rash is characteristically maculopapular
C foetal damage from the rubella virus can be prevented by gamma-globulin
D when vaccination is offered to school girls, prior serological tests are needed
E the posterior cervical glands are typically enlarged

32. The following diseases and types of genetic transmission are associated:

A Friedreich's ataxia — autosomal dominant
B sickle-cell disease — autosomal dominant
C dystrophia myotonica — x linked
D alpha$_1$-antitrypsin deficiency — autosomal recessive
E colour blindness — x linked

33. The following are recognised features of Wilson's disease:

A band keratitis
B low urinary copper
C liver disease resembling chronic active hepatitis
D reduced plasma caeruloplasmin
E osteomalacia

34. The following statements are true of attacks of acute intermittent porphyria (AIP):

A Ehrlich's aldehyde reagent is of value in diagnosis
B postural hypotension is a characteristic finding
C pain in the limbs is a characteristic complaint
D diazepam is a typical precipitant
E carbohydrate infusions are of value in management

35. In benign monoclonal gammopathy (monoclonal hypergammaglobulinaemia)

A there is a low level of serum albumin
B there is a marked increase in immature plasma cells in the bone marrow
C the 'M' band in the serum electrophoretic strip does not show a progressive rise over the course of time
D there is no anaemia
E there is no Bence-Jones protein in the urine

36. Recognised features of carotid artery stenosis include

A diplopia
B transient ipsilateral monocular blindness
C drop attacks
D a cervical bruit
E ipsilateral hemiplegia

37. Muscle pain may be due to

A steroid myopathy
B polyarteritis nodosa
C muscle phosphorylase deficiency (McArdle's disease)
D Guillain-Barré syndrome
E amyotrophic lateral sclerosis

38. In Bell's palsy

A the prognosis is worse if taste sensation is affected
B the prognosis is worse in infancy
C clonic facial spasm may be a complication
D perioral anaesthesia may be a feature
E inappropriate lacrimation characteristically occurs in the acute phase

39. There is a recognised association between autonomic neuropathy and

A parkinsonism
B infective polyneuropathy (Guillain-Barré)
C autosomal dominant mode of inheritance
D intussusception
E neurofibromatosis

40. A patient presents with a painful red eye. The following findings are more suggestive of anterior uveitis than acute conjunctivitis:

A blurring of vision
B profuse discharge
C small pupil
D photophobia
E clear media

41. Cystic fibrosis of the pancreas

A has an x-linked recessive inheritance
B is the commonest cause of chronic suppurative lung disease in children in the UK
C causes clubbing of the fingers
D produces sweat sodium concentrations over 80 mmol/l in the first 6 months of life
E can be diagnosed before birth by amniocentesis

42. In whooping cough

A occurrence is rare before 6 months of age
B subcutaneous (surgical) emphysema is a recognised complication
C there is a diagnostic complement fixation test
D there is a rapid and satisfactory recovery with erythromycin
E the chest X-ray is frequently normal

43. Recognised causes of stridor include

A foreign body in the left main bronchus
B *Haemophilus influenzae* infection
C vascular ring
D hypercalcaemia
E *C. diphtheriae* infection

44. A shift in the haemoglobin/oxygen dissociation curve to the right

A means that for a given pO_2 there is less oxygen per gram of haemoglobin
B occurs in anaemia
C occurs when the pCO_2 is increased
D could result from an increased concentration of 2,3 diphosphoglycerate in the erythrocytes
E is favoured by a fall in temperature

45. Hysterical amnesia

A typically is a patchy loss of memory
B typically resolves within 48 hours
C is a conscious reaction
D has a recognised association with head injury
E responds to abreaction

46. Recognised side-effects of lithium carbonate include

A polyuria
B hypopituitarism
C diarrhoea
D intention tremor
E hypothyroidism

47. The following are recognised associations of patients with calcium containing urinary stones:

A a positive family history
B a persistently low urinary pH
C hyperuricosuria
D small bowel malabsorption
E medullary-sponge kidney

48. Characteristic findings in minimal change glomerular disease include

A hypertension
B microscopic haematuria
C response to corticosteroids
D uraemia
E spontaneous remissions

49. On chest X-ray the upper zone is more commonly affected than the lower zone in

A asbestosis
B silicosis
C cryptogenic fibrosing alveolitis
D ankylosing spondylitis
E systemic sclerosis

50. Recognised causes of pulmonary eosinophilia (chest X-ray shadowing and peripheral blood eosinophilia) include

A *Ascaris lumbricoides* infestation
B systemic lupus erythematosus
C sarcoidosis
D polyarteritis nodosa
E cryptogenic fibrosing alveolitis

51. The following are typical features of Reiter's syndrome:

A balanitis circinata
B tenosynovitis
C a significantly raised frequency of HLA-B27
D symmetrical arthritis of the small joints of the hands
E retrobulbar neuritis

52. D-Penicillamine therapy in rheumatoid arthritis may

A reverse radiological erosive changes
B lower rheumatoid factor titres
C cause Goodpasture's syndrome
D produce ageusia (altered taste sensation)
E cause malabsorption

53. Osteoporosis

A frequently causes crush fractures of thoracic vertebrae but only rarely causes spinal cord compression
B may be diagnosed by a normal calcium and phosphate with raised alkaline phosphatase
C is characterised by the failure of matrix to calcify and form bone
D can cause secondary hyperparathyroidism
E can occur in a painful, localised form in the hand or foot following injury

54. A new assay has been developed for the measurement of plasma adrenaline. The following statements are correct:

A the coefficient of variation gives an idea of the sensitivity of the assay
B the accuracy of the assay is the degree to which repeated observations conform to each other
C the specificity of the assay is a reflection of the degree to which substances other than adrenaline interfere with the results
D the precision of the assay is an indication of the closeness of the measurement to their true value
E the sensitivity of the assay is related to the closeness that the lower limits of detection approximate to zero

55. The average heights of two groups of individuals are 1·48 metres and 1·85 metres respectively. The following tests might be useful in determining whether the differences between the groups were real or due to chance alone:

A Student's unpaired t-test
B Kendall rank correlation test
C Student's paired t-test
D Chi-square test
E Wilcoxon rank sums test

56. The following are features of atropine poisoning:

A fever
B bradycardia
C profuse sweating
D pin-point pupils
E hallucinations

57. In tropical sprue

A the incidence is greater amongst expatriate Caucasians in tropical areas than in the indigenous population
B the onset is usually insidious with diarrhoea and weight loss
C the condition can be differentiated from other causes of malabsorption by characteristic jejeunal biopsy appearances
D there may be a dramatic response to folic acid therapy alone in some cases
E macrocytic anaemia is nearly always present

58. The following are features of *Schistosoma haematobium* infestation:

A pruritus
B glomerulonephritis
C pulmonary hypertension
D successful response to trivalent arsenical drugs
E eosinophilia

59. The following are typical features of malaria due to *Plasmodium vivax:*

A recurrences due to hepatic infection
B severe haemolytic anaemia
C splenomegaly
D coma
E nephrotic syndrome

60. Amoebic liver abscess

A occurs typically in the left lobe
B may present 20 years or more after amoebic dysentery
C usually requires therapeutic needle aspiration
D characteristically causes jaundice
E is associated with a positive serological test in a majority of cases

End of Practice Exam

PRACTICE EXAM ANSWERS

1. **C E**

The median nerve enters the palm of the hand by passing deep to the flexor retinaculum and then supplies the muscles of the thenar eminence (but *not* the adductor pollicis), the first two lumbricals and digital branches to the thumb, index, middle and radial half of the ring finger. The median innervation of the first two lumbricals accounts for the index and middle fingers being less "clawed" than the ring and little fingers in an ulnar nerve palsy (i.e. there is preservation of the flexion of the M-P and of the extension of the interphalangeal joints).

2. **C E**

The metabolic acidosis of uraemia and diabetic ketoacidosis would make a high plasma bicarbonate an extremely unlikely occurrence. Most causes of hypokalaemia are associated with a metabolic alkalosis which can be gross in pyloric stenosis. In chronic cor pulmonale, a raised bicarbonate level would indicate renal compensation of a respiratory acidosis due to CO_2 retention.

3. **A B C**

Growth hormone raises the plasma phosphorus level which is not, however, a good index of disease activity in acromegaly. Hyperphosphataemia is believed to play an aetiological role in renal osteodystrophy, by leading to hyperparathyroidism. The plasma phosphorus is typically low in all vitamin D deficiency related bone disease. It is normal in Paget's disease.

4. **A B C E**

Oat cell lung cancers may secrete ADH. ADH released by blood volume contraction (See Q.167) contributes to the hyponatraemia of salt depletion and hyperglycaemia. Also, in dehydration, increased proximal tubular reabsorption limits the volume of fluid reaching the diluting segment of the distal tubule and hence water excretion. In hyperglycaemia, osmotically active solute in the blood also contributes to hyponatraemia. In hyperlipidaemia, hyponatraemia is more apparent then real, due to plasma water being replaced by sodium-free lipid.

5. None

The treatment of choice is intravenous heparin; the subcutaneous route is only appropriate for prophylaxis. The arterial pCO_2 and pO_2 are characteristically reduced. The chest X-ray is normal more often than not but may show areas of radiolucency due to oligaemia. There may also be vessel "cut off" and later, even without infarction, evidence of atelectasis.

6. A B

Complete and lesser degrees of A-V block are more common with posterior myocardial infarcts and characteristically resolve. This is probably related to the fact that the A-V node and Bundle of His are supplied by the right coronary artery in about 90% of cases. When complete heart block occurs with anterior infarcts it usually indicates massive necrosis, hence the poor prognosis. Chronic complete heart block is more often due to idiopathic sclerosis (Lenegre's disease) or fibrocalcific degeneration of the myocardium (Lev's disease) than to ischaemic heart disease.

7. None

Hyponatraemia and ankle oedema in these circumstances suggest secondary aldosteronism. Soft exudates indicate the accelerated phase of hypertension and a loin bruit suggests renal artery stenosis, in both of which conditions secondary aldosteronism occurs frequently. A loin bruit is not heard with Conn's tumours and there is no recognised association with thyroid disease.

8. B D

The majority of cases are secondary to bicuspid valves or of unknown aetiology. The sex incidence in these cases is predominantly male. The presence of mitral valve disease, significant aortic regurgitation or a female patient would suggest a rheumatic origin. Whilst the absence of a thrill generally indicates relatively mild disease, one may not be felt if the patient is obese, is in cardiac failure, or has emphysema. Patients may present in congestive cardiac failure rather than classically with dyspnoea, fatigue, angina or syncope, and in these circumstances the physical signs may be misleadingly unimpressive.

9. **B C E**

A murmur mimicking mitral stenosis may occur when there is greatly increased flow across a normal mitral valve in mitral regurgitation, VSD, patent ductus and occasionally in thyrotoxicosis and other hyperdynamic circulatory conditions. Similar murmurs occur in aortic regurgitation (Austin Flint) acute rheumatic fever (Carey Coombs) and with atrial myxomas. The murmur of tricuspid stenosis and tricuspid flow murmurs may occasionally be heard at the apex.

10. **A D E**

Nitrates act in angina mainly by reducing myocardial oxygen consumption through reducing aterial blood pressure and heart size (ventricular wall tension) by arterial and venous dilatation. Coronary artery dilatation is thought to occur only in individuals with normal coronary arteries. The fall in mean arterial pressure leads to a reflex increase in heart rate. In heart failure, the venodilator effect of nitrates predominates. (See Q.12)

11. **A D E**

The tetracyclines (except doxycycline) can aggravate uraemia dangerously and should be avoided in patients with anything other than minimal renal impairment. (See Q.33 Page 17) Penicillamine, like gold, produces an immune-complex glomerulonephritis. Cyclophosphamide can give a serious chemical cystitis.

12. **B D E**

Tricyclic antidepressants interfere with the neuronal uptake of adrenergic blocking drugs and prevent or reverse their hypotensive effects. Ephedrine, in the presence of a MAOI, can give dangerous hypertensive effects due to neurotransmitter release unmodified by monoamine oxidase. Tetracycline is not absorbed in the presence of iron (and magnesium, calcium and aluminium in antacid mixtures) due to the formation of insoluble complexes.

13. E

Morphine is detoxicated mainly by conjugation with glucuronic acid in the liver and should be used with caution in cirrhosis. Pin-point pupils (severe miosis) are an important sign of intoxication or addiction with opiates. Intestinal smooth muscle tone is increased and propulsive waves diminished, explaining the constipating effects of these drugs. The therapeutic effect of morphine in acute left ventricular failure is probably largely due to its venodilating action.

14. C D

Iodine is good preoperative treatment, but its concentration by the gland would be inhibited by perchlorate. Surgery carries several risks including hypoparathyroidism; this may occur transiently with spontaneous improvement and is rarely permanent. The concept of normocaleaemic latent hypoparathyroidism is now discredited. Radioiodine may induce thyroid cancer after administration in childhood but does not carry any significant risk of leukaemia. In a toxic adenoma the remaining normal thyroid tissue will have relatively suppressed iodine uptake reducing the risk of late hypothyroidism.

15. A C D

A family history may be obtained if the angioedema is part of an atopic diathesis when it is associated with urticaria. Hereditary angioedema is an autosomal dominant condition characterised by absence of functional C1-esterase inhibitor, involvement of the gastro-intestinal tract and potentially fatal attacks of upper respiratory obstruction. There is no urticaria.
A familial element to SLE is recognised but is not very strong.

16. A D E

Exfoliative dermatitis (erythroderma) will contribute to congestive cardiac failure by virtue of the increased blood flow in the skin, a factor also tending to *hypo-* not *hyper*thermia. Pruritus is common and not indicative of an underlying lymphoma.
Psoriasis is responsible for about 25% of cases of exfoliative dermatitis.
Lymphadenopathy is often marked with exfoliative dermatitis, constituting so-called dermatopathic lymphadenopathy.

17. A B C

The non-metastatic hypercalcaemia of malignancy cannot always be shown to be due to excess parathormone-like activity and in at least half the cases, responds to steroids. Human chorionic thyrotrophin found in the normal placenta and in chorioncarcinomas does not cause eye signs. Hypernephroma is a more frequent case of polycythaemia than phaeochromocytoma, cerebellar haemangiomata, uterine myomata and hepatomas. Ectopic ADH secretion presents with hyponatraemia and symptoms attributed to cerebral oedema. The myasthenic syndrome of malignancy (Eaton-Lambert) differs from classical myasthenia gravis in several respects including little or no response to neostigmine. Guanidine hydrochloride improves muscle strength in many of these patients.

18. A B D E

Other clinically important side-effects of phenothiazine therapy include orthostatic hypotension and the extra-pyramidal syndromes. (See Q.135)

19. B C E

The hypercalcaemia of hyperparathyroidism is often associated with raised parathormone (PTH) levels. A PTH level within the normal range however, is abnormal in the presence of hypercalcaemia, as the raised calcium should inhibit PTH. This occurs in the other causes of hypercalcaemia such as sarcoidosis. Hypercalciuria is not as great as would be predicted from other causes of hypercalcaemia, as there is increased renal tubular absorption of calcium. Foetal parathyroid activity may be suppressed by maternal hypercalcaemia, resulting in tetany in the neonate. A third of patients have hypertension, in part due to renal damage, but in some, recovering when hypercalcaemia is corrected. Over 80% of patients have a solitary adenoma, 15% have diffuse hyperplasia, and a small minority a carcinoma of one gland.

20. A D

Although chromophobe cells used to be considered non-secretory, this no longer is accepted and all anterior pituitary hormones including growth hormone have occasionally, but singly, been found in excess, Expansion of the pituitary fossa and extension to involve optic nerves, third, fourth and sixth cranial nerves and hypothalamus, may all occur, but curiously, the supraopticohypophyseal tract is invariably spared. There is an association with parathyroid hyperplasia or adenomas (MEA type 1, See Q.46 Page 24). Early in the course of the tumour there may only be evidence of gonadotrophin or thyrotrophin deficiency, but ultimately panhypopituitarism will develop.

21. A C D E

There are many other causes of salivary gland enlargement. These include mumps and other viral and non-viral infections, drugs such as guanethidine, phenylbutazone and iodides, malnutrition, cirrhosis and Sjögrens syndrome.

22. B D E

Spontaneous pain may be an early symptom in achalasia, often occurring after eating and due to spasm in the partially denervated oesophagus. Since there is failure of relaxation of the gastro-oesophageal sphincter, difficulty in swallowing liquids and solids occurs equally. Bolting food and emotional disturbances may be responsible for the initially intermittent dysphagia, so that malnutrition can be avoided early on in the course. Impact pain due to bolus obstruction in the oesophagus is a feature of organic stricture.

23. B D E

Acute pancreatitis may occur in hyperparathyroidism (and other hypercalcaemic conditions). Diffuse fibrosis without inflammation occurs in haemochromatosis. Mumps infections may involve the gland and, rarely, ascaria may enter the duct giving rise to acute pancreatitis. The passage of gallstones through the common bile duct is postulated to cause bile reflux into the pancreatic duct offering one explanation of the association with acute pancreatitis.

24. D E

Haemochromatosis may occur in alcoholic cirrhosis and be difficult to differentiate from the idiopathic hereditary form in which alcohol is not necessarily implicated. Hepatic pain may be a presenting feature. Although portal hypertension and liver failure may occur in the untreated patient, this happens less often than in Laennec's cirrhosis. Hepatoma occurs in over a third of treated patients and is the commonest cause of death. Phlebotomy, if carried out frequently enough, is as effective as chelating agents like desferrioxamine in depleting iron stores and thereby improving the prognosis.

25. None

The incubation period of gonorrhoea is from 2 to 8 days. The disease is far more prone to dissemination in women and when it does, characteristically gives fever, polyarthralgia, and necrotic skin lesions on the extremities (See Q.77). Local complications such as epididymitis and prostatitis, and, later, urethral stricture, are nowadays rare.

26. C D E

Almost every disease, bodily insult and drug has been credited with precipitating acute confusion. Commonly implicated factors are trauma, surgery, heart failure, infection, anoxia and sedative drugs. Confusion is not, however, a characteristic feature of myxoedema. Senile dementia is a very common predisposing condition and tricyclics may precipitate a confusional state. Non-hypotensive phenothiazines such as thioridazine may be used therapeutically but dealing with the precipitating factor is most important.

27. C

Classically, the bleeding time in haemophilia and Xmas disease is normal as these diseases do not affect the function of the skin vessels. In von Willebrand's disease, there is an abnormal bleeding time due to a deficiency of the von Willebrand factor in addition to a decreased level of factor VIII (See Q.90 and Q.100). Other causes of abnormal platelet-plug formation and a prolonged bleeding time, are severe thrombocytopenia, defects of platelet function and afibrinogenaemia.

28. B C D E

Radiotherapy is only useful for bone pain in myeloma. Poor renal function is closely correlated with a poor prognosis. Hyperviscosity occurs in IgA myeloma due to polymerisation of paraprotein molecules. Polyneuropathy occurs due to amyloidosis, or of unknown aetiology as with carcinoma.

29. A D E

Notification of infectious disease is obligatory under the Public Health Act 1968, and includes meningococcal meningitis, which can occur in epidemic form, measles which is highly infectious, and food poisoning which is multi-factorial. Actinomycosis is an endogenous disease, which is not spread from patient to patient. Aspergillosis, normally associated with *Aspergillus fumigatus* likewise is an endogenous infection, whereas *Aspergillus niger* is an ubiquitous fungus and can be spread by aerosol contamination, but is not normally considered a pathogen.

30. B C E

Legionnaire's disease caused by *Legionella pneumophilia,* a gram-negative bacillus, has been successfully treated with high dosage erythromycin often together with rifampicin.
Abnormal liver function tests are found in a large proportion of patients. Other common features are confusion, proteinuria and hyponatraemia. Epidemiologically, it has been associated with young men who are heavy drinkers and heavy smokers.

31. A E

The period of communicability for rubella is from about one week before to one week after the onset of the rash, or of other symptoms. The rash is characteristically macular. Foetal damage cannot be prevented by gammaglobulin but the extent of damage can be modified. By the time school girls are offered rubella vaccination about 50% already have rubella antibodies: it would be too expensive to screen all these girls and vaccinate only the sero-negative ones.

32. D E

Friedreich's ataxia and sickle-cell disease are both autosomal recessive disorders. Dystrophia myotonica has autosomal dominant inheritance and well illustrates features of dominant rather than recessive disorders. These are a late age of onset and a vaiable clinical picture. (See Q.209)

33. C D E

The basic abnormality in Wilson's disease is a failure to excrete copper into the bile. Excess copper is toxic and gives rise to various forms of liver disease, a neurological disorder affecting mainly the basal ganglia, Kayser-Fleischer rings in the cornea and renal tubular defects (hence the osteomalacia — See Q.191).
The plasma caeruloplasmin and total copper are reduced and the urinary copper excretion is high.

34. A B C E

Porphobilinogen excreted in large amounts in the urine in acute attacks gives a red colour with Ehrlich's reagent which is not extractable with chloroform (cf. urobilinogen and indoles). Labile hypertension, postural hypotension, tachycardia and neuritic limb pains are attributed to autonomic and peripheral nervous system dysfunction.
Classical precipitant drugs include barbiturates, anticonvulsants, oral contraceptives and sulphonamides. (See Q.34 Page 17)
Glucose infusions often help abort attacks.

35. C D E

In this condition, which may occur in as many as 3% of those over 70 years, there is an abnormal band of globulin present in the electrophoretic strip. Typically, the level of abnormal globulin (IgG in about 85% of cases) is under 30 g/l and the other serum proteins are normal. This condition is not associated with anaemia, abnormal numbers and types of plasma cells in the marrow, or the presence of Bence-Jones protein in the urine. A percentage have, however, developed multiple myeloma or lymphoma after many years of follow-up.

36. B D

Diplopia and drop attacks are brain stem symptoms and not likely to be the result of carotid artery stenosis.
Ipsilateral blindness may result because of embolisation of the ophthalmic artery. If the hemisphere is involved, the hemiplegia will be contralateral.

37. B C D E

Polyarteritis nodosa may lead to painful infarction of muscle. The glycogenoses, which lead to accumulation of lactate, as in myophosphorylase deficiency, are associated with pain in muscle on exercise.

In the Guillain-Barré syndrome, pain is a common presenting symptom before weakness and cutaneous sensory disturbance.

Painful contractions occur in spastic muscles in amyotrophic lateral sclerosis where lateral column degeneration is a major feature.

38. A C

The prognosis in Bell's palsy is worse in the elderly and with more proximal lesions which involve the chorda tympani and the nerve to stapedius. Facial spasm may occur in the early irritative phase and on recovery. (It also occurs in patients who have never had a Bell's palsy.) Gustatory lacrimation occurs on recovery due to anomalous regeneration of the seventh nerve fibres.

39. A B C

In idiopathic and post-encephalitic parkinsonism, the central sympathetic connections may degenerate. It is more extensive in the Shy-Drager syndrome.

It is increasingly recognised that autonomic neuropathy may complicate acute infective neuropathy, the most serious results being cardiac arrhythmias and postural hypotension. A familial form of autonomic neuropathy (Riley-Day syndrome) is recognised in children. It shows an autosomal dominant mode of inheritance.

40 A C D

Other causes of a 'red eye' are subconjunctival haemorrhage, which is not painful, and acute closed angle glaucoma and keratitis which are. With conjunctival injection, the vessels fade from fornix to limbus, and move with the conjunctiva. Ciliary vessel injection with intraocular inflammation gives the reverse findings. (See Q.137 and Q.138)

41. B C D

The inheritance of cystic fibrosis is by an autosomal recessive gene. Other causes of chronic suppurative lung disease such as bronchiectasis are quite rare now. A high sweat sodium (over 80 m mol/l) was originally thought *not* to occur in the first few months of life in these patients, but this has been disproved. Unfortunately, no prenatal diagnostic test, such as by amniocentesis, is yet available, though much research is proceeding towards this end. (See Q.73)

42. B E

Immunity to whooping cough is not transmitted trans-placentally to the foetus as it is with many other infectious diseases, and unfortunately, the disease is both frequent and serious to infants in the first six months. There is no satisfactory serological test, and diagnosis must rest on the clinical history and findings, blood count, and culture of the organism. Response to erythromycin is very uncertain and variable. In a few cases there may be chest X-ray changes showing patchy collapse, interstitial or surgical emphysema, but in the majority the X-ray is normal.

43. B C E

A foreign body in a main bronchus may cause initial spluttering and coughing when first inhaled, but will then probably be silent until infection or lung collapse occur. *Haemophilus influenzae* is a frequent secondary invader in acute laryngotracheitis, which causes marked stridor. A vascular ring round the trachea may cause definite, though rather faint stridor, and *C. diphtheriae* will cause stridor by infection of the fauces or larynx. (See Q.112)

44. A C D

The oxygen dissociation curve is usually plotted as the percentage saturation of haemoglobin with oxygen against oxygen tension. A shift to the right means that for a given oxygen tension there is reduced saturation of haemoglobin with oxygen. This shift can be brought about by an increase in hydrogen ion concentration, in pCO_2 and 2,3 diphosphoglycerate. The dissociation curve applies in anaemia even though the oxygen capacity is low.

45. A B D E

When amnesia is of hysterical origin, rather than due to some organic cause, emotionally charged events may be forgotten, whilst memory for other events taking place at the same time may be retained. The majority of such states resolve quickly as the situation which produced them alters. The symptoms are of subconscious, rather than conscious origin. The reaction can follow all kinds of traumatic events, but in particular, it is associated with head injury. The patient can be treated by being encouraged to release the emotion of the traumatic event by interview under light narcosis-abreaction.

46. A C E

Almost all patients taking lithium carbonate report polydipsia and polyuria, due to interference with ADH action in the kidney. A high serum lithium causes gastro-intestinal disturbances, weakness and fine tremor of the hands, but not an intention tremor. There is a risk of hypothyroidism in patients taking lithium, due to effects on intrathyroid iodine metabolism. (See Q.31)

47. A C D E

There is a marked tendency for idiopathic hypercalciuria, which is a predominantly male disease and the commonest single cause of calcium stones, to run in families. Persistently acid urine is a feature of uric acid stone formers. Calcium phosphate tends to precipitate in alkaline urine whereas calcium oxalate stones do not depend on urine pH. Factors that predispose to oxalate stones include hyperuricosuria either dietary or due to gout and increased absorption of oxalate from the bowel in malabsorption states.

48. C E

This condition gives a "pure" nephrotic syndrome without features of acute nephritis such as hypertension, uraemia or haematuria. Microscopic haematuria is, however, found in an appreciable minority of cases and on occasions severe uraemia occurs due to pre-renal factors and tubular obstruction. Remissions and relapses are highly characteristic. The former can be spontaneous due to intercurrent infection or corticosteroid therapy.

49. B D

Pulmonary fibrosis of silicosis and ankylosing spondylitis affects predominantly the upper zones whereas that of asbestosis, fibrosing alveolitis and systemic sclerosis occurs predominantly in the lower zones. In systemic sclerosis there may be a combination of diffuse fibrosis and basal aspiration pneumonia.

50. A D

Perhaps the most important cause of pulmonary eosinophilia in the UK is allergic broncho-pulmonary aspergillosis, which can lead to severe lung damage. Other causes include allergic reactions to a variety of parasites such as filaria, (tropical eosinophilia) or drugs (nitrofurantoin, sulphonamides, chlorpropamide, and others). Loeffler's syndrome is a term used to describe mild transient illnesses with pulmonary eosinophilia for which no cause is found.

51 A C

Although tendinitis (e.g. Achilles, plantar fasciitis) is common, tenosynovitis is more suggestive of gonococcal disease. (See Q.77) Reiter's arthritis is typically asymetrical and affects the weight-bearing joints of the lower limbs, including the small joints of the feet and the sacro-iliac joints. In addition to the classical conjunctivitis, anterior uveitis is a frequent and important occurrence.

52. B C D

There is reasonable, but not conclusive, evidence that only one drug can cause radiological reversal of erosions, and that is gold. Like gold, penicillamine can lower rheumatoid factor titres in parallel with a reduction in the activity of the disease. The recorded side effects are legion: commonly rash and pruritus, ageusia (a blunting of taste perception which is not dose related), leucopenia, thrombocytopenia and proteinuria secondary to an immune complex nephritis. Rarer penicillamine-induced syndromes include myasthenia gravis, SLE, polymyositis, thyroiditis, haemolytic anaemia and Goodpasture's syndrome.

53. A E

The characteristic biochemical pattern is of normal calcium, phosphate and alkaline phosphatase. A raised phosphatase would suggest a recent fracture or osteomalacia which can occur in the presence of normal calcium and phosphate.
Osteoporosis is a reduction of bone tissue per unit volume of anatomical bone — it has a normal composition. In osteomalacia there is failure of matrix to calcify and form bone giving the histological appearance of widened osteoid seams. Painful localised osteoporosis in the extremities is known as Sudek's atrophy or algodystrophy.

54. C E

The coefficient of variation of the assay is an indication of the degree to which repeated measurements conform to each other, i.e. it is an index of reproducibility or precision. The accuracy is the closeness of the measurements to their true values. The specificity of the adrenaline assay reflects the degree to which substances other than adrenaline interfere with the results — e.g. a completely specific assay measures adrenaline and nothing else.

55. A E

Student's paired t-test might be used to compare the height of one group on two separate occasions. The Kendall rank correlation test might be used to relate height to another variable, such as weight or age.
Chi-square tests are used for determining whether observed frequencies in a distribution differ significantly from the frequencies which might be expected according to some assumed hypothesis.

56. A E

Atropine poisoning produces parasympathetic blockade and a toxic psychosis characterised by mania, hallucinations and delirium. There is dry mouth, dilated pupils, a dry, flushed skin, fever, tachycardia, urinary retention and abdominal distension. Atropine-like drugs used for Parkinsonism and gastro-intestinal disorders can give the same picture.

57. A D E

The onset of tropical sprue is usually abrupt. The greater incidence in expatriates than in the indigenous population is cited as evidence in favour of an infective cause. The appearances of partial villous atrophy seen on jejeunal biopsy are non-specific. Remission may follow folic acid therapy alone, although broad spectrum antibiotics are usually also given. Macrocytic anaemia may be the only deficiency manifest.

58. A B C E

Pruritic dermatitis is an early and may be the only manifestation of a schistosomal infestation. In addition to the major urinary tract complications of severe, fibrosing inflammatory changes, an immune-complex glomerulonephritis occurs, and can lead to the nephrotic syndrome. Eggs can reach the lungs and give obstructive changes in the pulmonary circulation. The classical drugs used in schistosomiasis are trivalent antimonials, but niridazole (Ambilhar) is as effective and less toxic.

59. A C

Persistent hepatic infection with *P. vivax* (and *P. ovale*) can give clinical recurrences years after the initial infection. Severe haemolysis and coma are found in *P. falciparum* infections and the nephrotic syndrome occurs mainly in children with *P. malariae.*

60. B E

The commonest site of a solitary amoebic liver abscess is the upper part of the right lobe. Jaundice only occurs with multiple or very large abscesses. Therapeutic (and/or diagnostic) needle aspiration is required for only a minority of cases in the UK, thanks to effective diagnostic techniques and drugs.